Ophthalmology Com

Ophthalmology Companion

Wilhelm Happe and Jakob Daniel Fischel

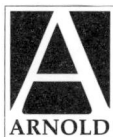

ARNOLD

A member of the Hodder Headline Group
LONDON • SYDNEY • AUCKLAND

Co-published in the USA by
Oxford University Press, Inc., New York

First English language edition published in Great Britain in 1998 by
Arnold, a member of the Hodder Headline Group,
338 Euston Road, London NW1 3BH
http://www.arnoldpublishers.com

Original German language edition – *Memorix Augenheilkunde*
© 1996 Chapman & Hall Gmbh D-69469 Weinheim, Germany

English translation © 1998 Arnold

Co-published in the United States of America by
Oxford University Press Inc.,
198 Madison Avenue, New York, NY10016
Oxford is a registered trademark of Oxford University Press

Whilst the advice and information in this book are believed to be true and
accurate at the date of going to press, neither the author nor the publisher
can accept any legal responsibility or liability for any errors or omissions
that may be made. In particular (but without limiting the generality of the
preceding disclaimer) every effort has been made to check drug dosages;
however, it is still possible that errors have been missed. Furthermore,
dosage schedules are constantly being revised and new side-effects
recognized. For these reasons the reader is strongly urged to consult the
drug companies' printed instructions before administering any of the drugs
recommended in this book.

Some drugs and medical devices presented in this publication have FDA
clearance for limited use in restricted research settings. It is the
responsibility of the health care provider to ascertain the FDA status of
each drug or device planned for use in their clinical practice.

British Library Cataloguing in Publication Data
A catalogue record for this book is available from the British Library

Library of Congress Cataloging-in-Publication Data
A catalog record for this book is available from the Library of Congress

ISBN 0 340 74093 0

1 2 3 4 5 6 7 8 9 10

Typeset in 9/10 Plantin by Best-set Typesetters Ltd, Hong Kong
Printed and bound in Great Britain by the Alden Press, Oxford

What do you think about this book? Or any other Arnold title?
Please send your comments to feedback.arnold@hodder.co.uk

CONTENTS

PREFACE

This book was first published in German in 1996 in the Memorix series. It deals with common as well as various uncommon ophthalmic and ophthalmic-related diseases. However, it is not meant to replace an ophthalmic textbook, but rather to serve as a handy reference during clinical situations such as during a busy clinic. The content has been chosen to reflect generally accepted practices in the classifications, diagnostic procedures, differential diagnostic strategies and therapeutic practices.

Wilhelm Happe
Department of Strabismology and Neuro-ophthalmology
University Eye Hospital
Robert Koch Strasse 40
D-37075 Gottingen
Germany

It was my honour and pleasure to be the translator and co-author of the English edition of this book, which is designed to support ophthalmologists at all levels. Its numerous illustrations and problem-oriented tables will hopefully provide quick answers to specific problems.

Grateful thanks are due to Mr A B Tullo and Miss J Ashworth of the Royal Manchester Eye Hospital, who reviewed and commented upon this English edition.

Jakob Daniel Fischel
London
U.K.

ABBREVIATIONS

AC: **A**nterior **c**hamber
ANA: **A**nti-**n**uclear **a**ntibodies
CL: **C**ontact **l**ens
cm/m: Prism dioptre
CNS: **C**entral **n**ervous **s**ystem
CT: **C**omputed **t**omography
DD: **D**isc **d**iameter
DR: **D**iabetic **r**etinopathy
EOG: **E**lectro-**o**culography
ERG: **E**lectro**r**etinography
IOP: **I**ntraocular **p**ressure
MRI: **M**agnetic **r**esonance **i**maging
PDR: **P**roliferative **d**iabetic **r**etinopathy
RPE: **R**etinal **p**igment **e**pithelium
VF: **V**isual **f**ield

FUNDAMENTALS

SI UNITS

	Name of unit	Symbol	Equivalent
Length	metre	**m**	
Area	square metre	**m²**	
Volume	cubic metre	**m³**	$= 1000\,dm^3 = 10001$
	litre	**l**	
Weight	kilogram	**kg**	
Amount of substance	moles	**mol**	
Molarity	moles per cubic metre	**mol/m³**	$= 10^3\,mol/l$
Catalytic activity	katal	**kat**	$= mol/s$
Power	newton	**N**	$= 0.102\,kgp$ (kgf)
Unit of power	watt	**W**	$=$ **J/s**
Energy	joule	**J**	$= 0.239\,cal_{th}$
	kilojoule	**kJ**	$= 0.239\,kcal_{th}$
Thermodynamic	kelvin	**K**	$1\,K = 1°C$
temperature	celsius	**°C**	$0°C = 273.15\,K$
Pressure	pascal	**Pa**	$= 0.0075\,mmHg$ (Torr)
	kilopascal	**kPa**	$= 7.5\,mmHg$ (Torr)
	bar	bar	$= 100\,\mathbf{kPa}\ (10^5\,\mathbf{Pa})$
	physical atmosphere	atm	$= 101.3\,\mathbf{kPa}$
Speed	metre	**m/s**	
Acceleration	metres per second²	**m/s²**	
Frequency	hertz	**H_z**	
Electric current	ampère	**A**	
Electric load	coulomb	**C**	
Electric potential	volt	**V**	
Electric capacity	farad	**F**	
Electrical resistance	ohm	**Ω**	
Electrical conductance	siemens	**S**	
Luminous intensity	candela	**cd**	
Illumination	lux	**lx**	
Wavelength	Ångström	**Å**	$= 0.1\,nm = 10^{-10}\,m$
Radioactivity	becquerel	**Bq**	$= 0.27 \times 10^{-10}\,Ci$
	(previously Curie)	(Ci)	$= 2.7 \times 10^{10}\,\mathbf{Bq}$

	Name of unit	Symbol	Equivalent
Absorbed dosage	gray	**Gy**	$= 100 \, rd$
	(previously rad)	(rd)	$= 0.01 \, \textbf{Gy}$
Exposure	röntgen	R	$= 2.58 \times 10^{-4} \, \textbf{C/kg}$
Equivalent doses	sievert	Sv	$= 100 \, rem$
	(previously rem)	(rem)	$= 0.01 \, Sv$

BIOSTATISTICS

	Cohort	**Patient**	**Normal**
Test:	Positive	True positive (TP) **Sensitivity**	False positive (FP)
	Negative	False negative (FN)	True negative (TN) **Specificity**

TESTS ARE DEFINED BY:

Specificity $\dfrac{TN}{FP + TN}$ Sensitivity $\dfrac{TP}{TP + FN}$

STANDARD NORMAL DISTRIBUTION

(characteristic 'bell-shaped' symmetrical curve)

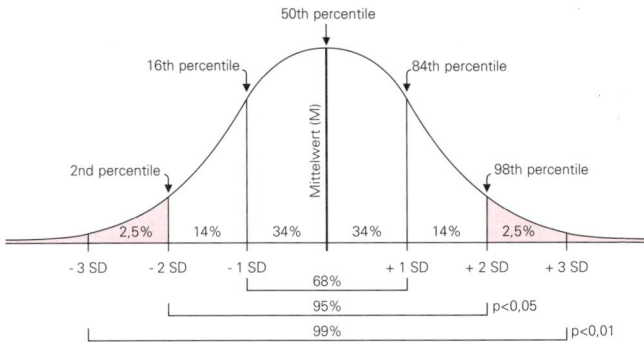

$M \pm 2$ standard deviations (SD) = 95% of values in normal subjects

Mean $(M) = x/n$; $x =$ total of values; $n =$ number of items

SEM (standard error of the mean) $= \dfrac{SD}{\sqrt{n}}$

Null hypothesis (H_0)	**True**	**False**
Rejection	Type I error ($P = \alpha$)	No error ($1 - \alpha$)
Acceptance	No error ($1 - \beta$)	Type II error ($P = \beta$)

EPIDEMIOLOGY

EPIDEMIOLOGICAL TERMS

Incidence: The number of newly diagnosed cases of a certain disease per year per 100 000 inhabitants

Prevalence: The number of cases of a certain disease per year per 100 000 inhabitants

Mortality: The number of deaths from a certain disease per year per 100 000 inhabitants

Lethality: The number of deaths from a certain disease per number of newly affected subjects

CRITERIA OF MEDICAL MEASUREMENTS

Objectivity: Do different examiners achieve similar results?

Reliability: Do repeated measurements under the same conditions achieve identical results?

Validity: Are the assessed variables really the ones that should be measured?

GENETICS

PEDIGREE SYMBOLS

□ Unaffected male	□○ Non-identical twins	
○ Unaffected female	○○ Identical twins	
⊡ Examined subject	● Miscarriage	
□○ Parents	◇ Unknown whether male or female	
□○ Consanguinity	■ Affected male	
□○□□ Siblings	◪ Heterozygous	

OCULAR MEASUREMENTS

Eyelids

Length of lid fissure	9 mm
Width of lid fissure	28–30 mm
Length of upper lid tarsus	25 mm
Height of upper lid tarsus	9–10 mm
Height of lower lid tarsus	4–5 mm

Globe	Sagittal diameter	24 mm
	Keratofoveal distance	23.5 mm (newborns 16 mm)
	Equatorial circumference	75 mm
	Weight	7 g
	Volume	6.5 ml
Extra-ocular muscles	Limbus/insertion distance	
	• medial rectus	5.5 mm/10.2 mm
	• lateral rectus	6.9 mm/9.4 mm
	• superior rectus	7.7 mm/10.1 mm
	• inferior rectus	6.5 mm/8.6 mm
	• superior oblique	14 mm/11 mm
	• inferior oblique	18 mm/10 mm
Lacrimal system	Secretion rate	2.4 µl/min
	Volume of tear film	6.5 µl
	Tear film thickness	7 µm
	pH value of tear film	7.4 (7.3–7.7)
Cornea	Diameter	
	• adults	Vertical 10.5 mm
		Horizontal 11.5 mm
	• first year of life	Horizontal 9.5–10 mm (definitely hydrophthalmos if >12 mm)
	Thickness	Centre 0.5 mm
		Periphery 0.7 mm
	Endothelial cell count (central)	Newborn 4000 cells/mm^2
		Adult 2000 cells/mm^2
	Refractive power	43 dpt centrally
	Radius of curvature	7.8 mm centrally (anterior surface)
	Refractive index	13.7
Sclera	Thickness	
	• limbal	0.8 mm
	• equatorial	0.5 mm
	• under and anterior to the recti insertion	0.3 mm
	Sites of perforation of the vortex veins	20–22 mm above the limbus
		18–19 mm below the limbus
Lens	Sagittal diameter	
	• newborn	3.5 mm
	• 2–5th decade	4 mm
	• 8–9th decade	5 mm
	Refractive power	19–33 dpt
	Refractive index	1.42
	Thickness of lens capsule	Anterior pole 8–14 µm
		Equator 7–17 µm
		Posterior pole 2–4 µm
	Lens fibres	Length 8–12 mm
		Thickness 4–6 µm
		Total number of fibres 2100–2300

Anterior/ posterior chamber	Volume of anterior chamber	140–230 mm^3
	Anterior chamber depth	3 mm
	Volume of posterior chamber	60 mm^3
Aqueous humour	Production rate	2–3 μl/min
	Diameter of Schlemm's canal	0.4 mm
	Average intra-ocular pressure	15 mmHg
	Normal episcleral venous pressure	10 mmHg
Iris	Total diameter	12 mm
	Pupillary diameter	1–9 mm
	Width of sphincter pupillae	0.5–1 mm
Ciliary body	Width of pars plana	4 mm
	Width of pars plicata	2 mm
	Number of ciliary processes	70–80
	Length of ciliary process	2 mm
	Thickness of ciliary process	0.5 mm
	Height of ciliary process	0.8–1 mm
	Distance from ora serrata to scleral spur	
	• temporal	7.5–8 mm
	• nasal	6.5–7 mm
Choroid	Total thickness	
	• fundal	0.2–0.3 mm
	• equator	0.1–0.15 mm
	Thickness of Bruch's membrane	1–3 μm
	Diameter of chorio-capillary vessels	8–20 μm
	Diameter	
	• of larger arterioles	50–100 μm
	• of smaller veins	10–40 μm
	• of veins	20–100 μm
Retina	Number of rods	120 million
	Number of cones	6 million
	Distance from limbus to ora serrata	6.5–7.5 mm
	Distance from ora serrata to equator	5–6 mm
Macula	Distance from centre of optic disc to foveola	4.2 mm (15°)
	Macular diameter	5 mm horizontal
	Foveal diameter	1.5 mm
	Diameter of the avascular foveolar zone	0.5 mm
	Foveolar diameter	0.35 mm
Vitreous	Volume	4 mm
	Specific weight	1.005–1.009
Optic disc and optic nerve	Horizontal papillary diameter	1.7 mm (6°)
	Distance from limbus to optic disc	27 mm nasally
		31 mm temporally
	Optic nerve length	35–55 mm (optic disc to chiasma)
	Optic nerve diameter	Intra-orbital 3–4 mm
		Intra-cranial 4–7 mm

Note: Values may vary. The above are averages.

BLOOD TESTS

BLOOD COUNT

Haematocrit	Women	35–47%	
	Men	40–52%	
Erythrocytes	Women	3.8–5.2 million/µl	
	Men	4.4–5.9 million/µl	
Haemoglobin	Women	12–16 g/dl	7.4–9.9 mmol/l
	Men	13–18 g/dl	8.1–11.2 mmol/l
Thrombocytes		150 000–400 000/µl	
Leukocytes	Adults	4 000–9 000/µl	
	Children	5 000–75 000/µl	

BLOOD PLASMA

Total protein	6–8.5 g/dl	60–85 g/l
Albumin	3.5–5.0 g/dl	35–50 g/l
Total bilirubin	0.3–1.0 mg/dl	5–17 µmol/l
Creatinine	0.6–1.5 mg/dl	60–130 µmol/l
Sodium	135–145 mEq/l	135–140 mmol/l
Potassium	3.5–5.0 mEq/l	3.5–5.0 mmol/l
Calcium	8.5–10.6 mg/dl	2.2–2.7 mmol/l
Glucose	70–110 mg/dl	4.0–6.0 mmol/l
Urea	15–40 mg/dl	2.5–6.7 mmol/l
Uric acid	3.0–7.0 mg/dl	180–420 µmol/l
Cholesterol	140–250 mg/dl	3.6–6.4 mmol/l
Triglyceride	50–250 mg/dl	0.6–3.0 mmol/l
Folic acid	6–15 mg/dl	14–34 mmol/l

COAGULATION

Partial thromboplastin time, also called KCCT (kaolin cephalin clotting time)	30–40 s
Plasma thrombin time	18–24 s (2–3-fold decrease in maximum heparinization)
Thromboplastin time	70–120% (10–20% is therapeutic range in oral anticoagulation
Fibrinogen	150–450 mg/dl

Oral anticoagulation is monitored using the INR = International Normalized Ratio (ratio of prothrombin time compared with control) Normal range = 0.9–1.2

INFLAMMATORY PARAMETERS

Erythrocyte sedimentation rate (ESR)*	Men	after 1 h: 3–8 mm
		after 2 h: 5–18 mm
	Women	after 1 h: 6–11 mm
		after 2 h: 6–20 mm

*Usually the Westergren method is used   Men: age in years ÷ 2
Women: (age in years + 10) ÷ 2

Eosinophil granulocytes	2–4% (collagen, parasitic and allergic diseases)
C3 complement	55–120 mg/dl (collagen diseases, temporal arteritis)
C4 complement	20–50 mg/dl (collagen diseases, temporal arteritis)
C-reactive protein	<1.0 mg/dl

SLIT LAMP EXAMINATION

FORMS OF ILLUMINATION WITH THE SLIT LAMP (BIOMICROSCOPE)

Diffuse illumination

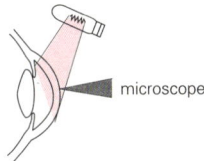

microscope

Direct illumination

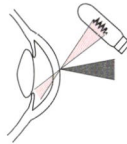

Indirect illumination

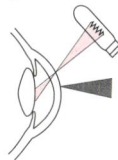

Retro-illumination

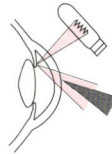

Specular reflection

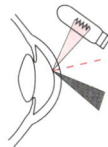

Scleral scatter

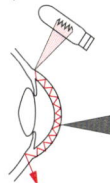

STATIC (AUTOMATED) PERIMETRY

POSSIBLE STIMULUS RESPONSES

		Stimulus	
		Present	Absent
Response	Seen	True positive (sensitivity)	False positive
	Not seen	False negative	True negative (specificity)

DEFINITION OF DECIBELS

Decibel is a unit used to express relative difference in power, equal to ten times the common logarithm ($\log_{10}$) of the ratio of the two levels. In perimetry, a decibel (dB) scale is a logarithmic scale where 10 dB = 1 log unit

$$E \text{ (dB)} = 10 \log (L_{max}/L)$$

E difference in light sensitivity
L_{max} maximum luminance intensity (cd/m²), dependent on machine used
L stimulus luminance intensity (cd/m²)

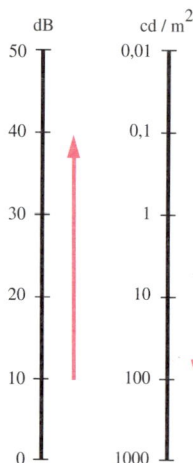

dB	cd/m²
50	0,01
40	0,1
30	1
20	10
10	100
0	1000

VISUAL FIELD INDEXES

Common terminology
Mean defect (MD)
Pattern standard deviation (PSD)
Corrected pattern standard deviation (CPSD)
Loss variance (LV)
Corrected loss variance (CLV)
Short-term fluctuation (SF)
Long-term fluctuation (LF)

Systematic terminology
Global mean (GM)
Global standard deviation (GS)
Global standard deviation corrected (GSC)
Global variance (GV)
Global variance corrected (GVC)
Global short-term fluctuation (GSF)
Global long-term fluctuation (GLF)

QUANTIFICATION OF VISUAL FIELD DATA

Visual field data are usually presented in a graphical format, as a visual field chart. However, the data presented in the field chart can be reduced to numbers which represent certain features of the visual field data (quantification).

Quantification allows the **rate** of progressive field loss to be monitored more objectively. It also enables **comparison** of individual results with those of a normal population (genuine visual field defects can be distinguished from field defects which may be normal, e.g. for the patient's age).

Topographical format

Loss variation

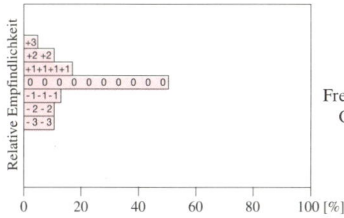

Frequency Curve

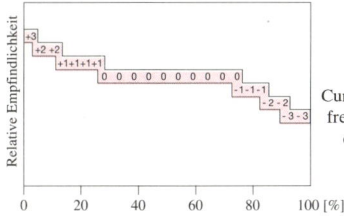

Cumulative frequency curve

SENSITIVITY OF AUTOMATED PERIMETRY

Absolute sensitivity	Threshold (dB)
Relative sensitivity	Deviation from age-related and locality-related data
Individual sensitivity	Individual deviation

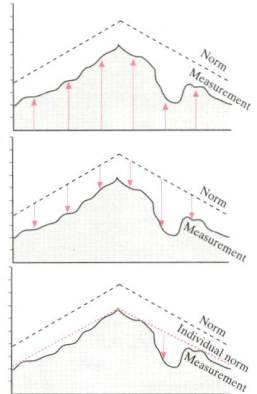

KINETIC PERIMETRY

GOLDMANN PERIMETER: EXAMINATION TECHNIQUE

Background luminance intensity	$1 \, cd/m^2$ ($=3.14 \, asb$)
Bowl radius	33 cm
Correction in cases of presbyopia	3 dpt

Stimulus	V_4, I_4, I_3, I_2, I_1
Stimulus movement	1–2°/s
Distance of meridians	15–30°
Examination of the blind spot	I_2

GOLDMANN PERIMETER: STANDARDIZED PARAMETERS

Target size	0	I	II	III	IV	V
Nominal size (30 cm distance)	$0.06\,mm^2$	$0.25\,mm^2$	$1\,mm^2$	$4\,mm^2$	$16\,mm^2$	$64\,mm^2$
Visual angle (mean angle)	~3′ (0.05°)	~6′ (0.11°)	~12′ (0.22°)	~24′ (0.43°)	~48′ (0.86°)	~100′ (1.72°)

Goldmann filter	Log/decibel scale (intervals of 0.1 log units = 1 dB)	Goldmann stimulus (intervals of 0.5 = log units = 5 dB)	Luminance intensity [apostilb]	Luminance intensity [candela/m^2]
a	0.40	1	31.4	10
b	0.50	2	100	31.4
c	0.63	3	314	100
d	0.79	4	1000	314 (absolute loss)
e	1.00 (usual position)	[asb] = [cd/m^2]		

COLOURED STIMULI (COLOUR ISOPTERS)

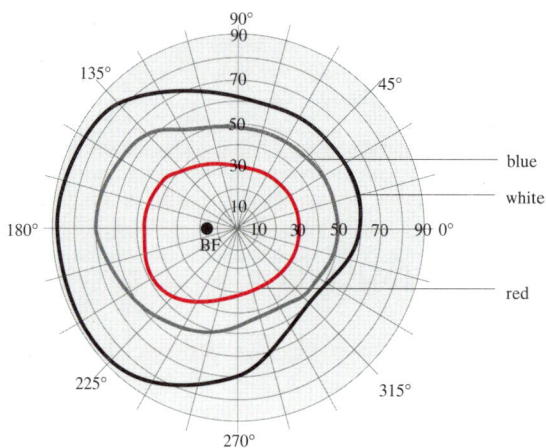

FLUORESCEIN ANGIOGRAPHY

PHENOMENA IN FLUORESCEIN ANGIOGRAPHY

Functional phenomena

Normal	Pathology	Example
Dense retinal capillaries (inner blood–retinal barrier)	Endothelial leaks	Diabetic retinopathy
	Zonulae occludentes defects (unclosed spaces between the endothelial cells)	Inflammations
	Defects in vessel walls	Proliferations
Choroidal capillaries contain multiple fenestrations through which fluorescein molecules that are not bound to albumin leak into the extravascular space	Focal permeability increased	Inflammations
Intact RPE (outer blood–retinal barrier)	Focal barrier breakdown	Central serous retinopathy

Mechanical phenomena

Normal	Pathology	Example
Strong adhesion between RPE and Bruch's membrane	Hemidesmosome disruption	Separation between the RPE and Bruch's membrane (RPE detachment); subretinal neovascularizations

Optical phenomena

Normal	Pathology	Example
Neuroretina is transparent	Reduced transparency	Oedema
RPE is not fully transparent (melanin deposition)	Pigmentary Shift Dehiscence	Hyaline deposits, scarring, areolar degeneration, RPE tear (physiological in the fovea), pigment epithelium hyperplasia

Normal	Pathology	Example
Bruch's membrane is semi-transparent	Dehiscence	Angioid streaks, traumatic ruptures, myopic lacquer cracks
Diffuse choroidal fluorescence (the capillaries of the choroid form a tight meshwork of channels with little extravascular space)	Hypofluorescence despite preserved transparency of the superimposed layers	Naevi, melanomas (own vessels)

Static and kinetic phenomena

Pathology
Stenoses
Dilatations
Aneurysms
Nonperfusion zones
Collaterals
Neovascularizations

DIFFERENTIAL DIAGNOSIS OF HYPOFLUORESCENCE

1. Blocked fluorescence (masking)

- of the retinal fluorescence — Opacity
  - of the anterior media
  - of the inner retinal layers

- of the choroidal fluorescence — Opacity
  - of the deep retinal layers
  - of the RPE
  - of Bruch's membrane
  - of the choroid

2. Vascular filling defects

- of the retinal vessels — Arteries
  Veins
  Capillaries

- of the optic nerve vessels — Capillaries

- of the choroidal vessels — Physiological
  Occlusion of the posterior ciliary arteries
  Choroidal tissue loss

DIFFERENTIAL DIAGNOSIS OF HYPERFLUORESCENCE

1. **Autofluorescence**
   (pre-injection photographs)

   Hyaline deposits in optic nerve
   Astrocytoma

2. **Window defect**
   (caused by RPE atrophy which
   produces increased visibility of the
   underlying choroidal fluorescence)

   Congenital reduced pigmentation
   (e.g. physiological, myopia, albinism)
   Atrophy (inflammatory, toxic,
   ischaemic, traumatic)

3. **Anomalous vessels**
   - of the retina and optic disc

     Neovascularization
     Vascular tortuousity, dilatation
     Anastomoses
     Aneurysms
     Tumour vessels
     Hamartoma

   - of the choroid

     Subretinal neovascularization
     Tumour vessels
     Hamartoma

4. **Leakage**
   - in a pre-formed space (pooling)

     Cystoid oedema
     RPE detachment

   - in a tissue (staining)

     Retinal (not cystoid) oedema
     Hyaline deposits (sub-retinal)

ASPECTS OF ASSESSING FLUORESCEUCE ANGIOGRAMS

Affected system	Manifestation
Retinal vascular architecture	Vascular occlusion
	Anomalies
	Neovascularizations
Blood–retinal barrier	Leakage
Abnormal transparency	Reduced transparency (masking hypofluorescence)
	Defects (hyperfluorescence)
Haemodynamics	Delayed vascular filling
	Retrograde vascular filling

Note: Nausea, vomiting, itching, skin rash, less frequently bronchospasm and rarely anaphylactic shock and acute pulmonary oedema may occur as side-effects of fluorescein injection. According to hospital emergency treatment regulations, adequate amounts of antihistamines, corticosteroids, adrenaline derivatives etc should be administered.

ELECTRO-DIAGNOSIS

ANATOMICAL STRUCTURES AND CORRESPONDING ELECTROPHYSIOLOGICAL TEST

Neuroretina

Photoreceptors	ERG: a-wave
Bipolar cells, Müller's cells	ERG: b-wave
Interneurone cells (amakrine cells)	Oscillatory potentials
Ganglion cells	Pattern ERG
Pigment epithelium	EOG (ERG)
Optic nerve	VEP, ERG

RETINAL DISORDERS AND ELECTROPOTENTIALS ACCORDING TO LAYER

- Myambutol intoxication
- Glaucoma

- Retinoschisis
- X-chromosome linked night blindness

b-wave   ERG

a-wave

- Digitalis (digoxin) intoxication
- Cone dystrophy
- Retinitis pigmentosa
- Stargardt's macular dystrophy
- Best's vitelliform macular dystrophy
- Central areolar choroidal dystrophy
- Choroideremia
- Gyrate atrophy

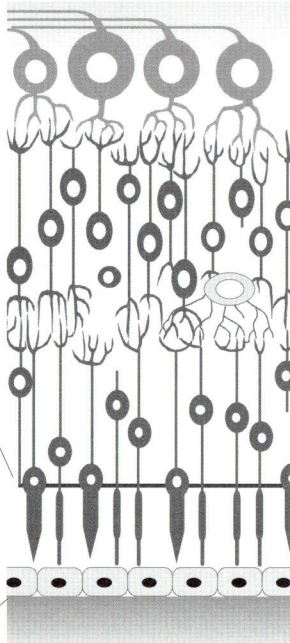

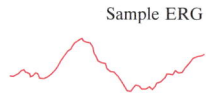

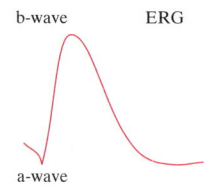

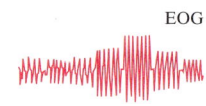

Sample ERG

EOG

ELECTRORETINOGRAPHY (ERG)

MINIMAL EXTENT OF AN ELECTRORETINOGRAPHIC INVESTIGATION (ACCORDING TO THE INTERNATIONAL SOCIETY OF CLINICAL ELECTROPHYSIOLOGY IN VISION)

[Marmor MF, Arden GB, Nilsson SEG, Zrenner E (1989) Standard for clinical electroretinography. *Arch Ophthalmol* **107**:816–819]

Dark-adapted:

Cone response

0.0096 cds/m^2

200 µV · 50 ms

Maximal response (rods–cones)

2.4 cds/m^2

200 µV · 50 ms

Oscillatory potentials

2.4 cds/m^2

40 µV · 50 ms

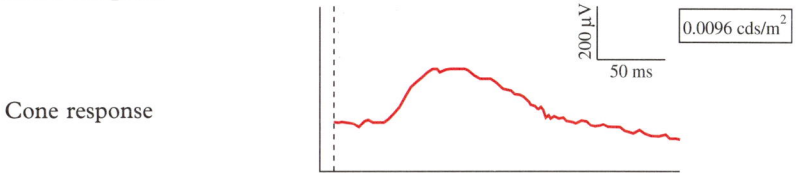

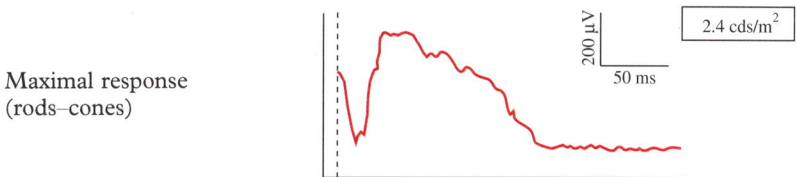

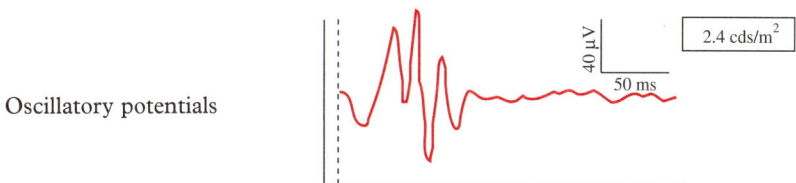

Light-adapted:

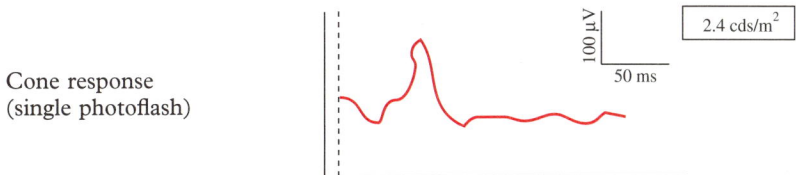

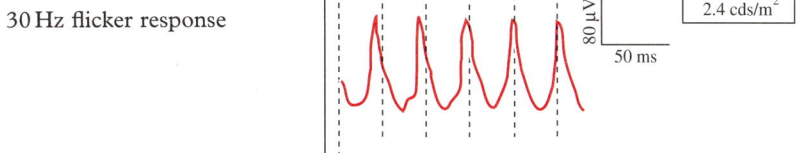

Cone response (single photoflash)

2.4 cds/m^2

100 µV · 50 ms

30 Hz flicker response

2.4 cds/m^2

80 µV · 50 ms

ELECTRO-OCULOGRAPHY (EOG)

NORMAL ELECTRO-OCULOGRAM

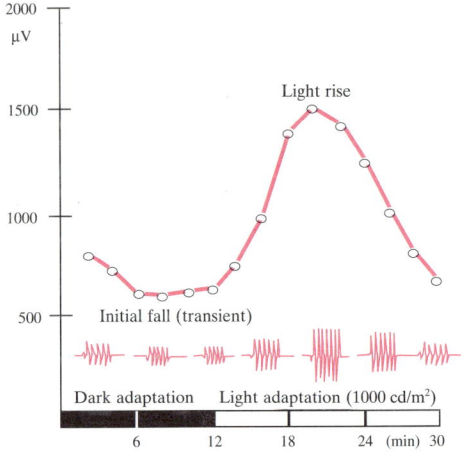

EOG IS INDICATED IN:

Suspected diagnosis
Best's vitelliform macular dystrophy
Carrier identification in Best's dystrophy
Treatment monitoring (e.g.
  phenothiazines, chloroquine)
Tapetoretinal degenerations

Comment
Absent light peak
Genetic counselling
EOG in addition to colour vision
  testing, and ERG
EOG indicated if ERG not
  available

$$\text{Arden ratio} = \frac{\text{Average of six readings taken at the 'light peak'}}{\text{Average of six readings taken at the 'dark trough'}} \times 100\%$$

EVALUATION OF THE ARDEN RATIO

Normal	>180%
Probably normal	180–165%
Subnormal	165–130%
Pathological	130–110%
Extinct	<110%
Inverted	EOG falls with light

COLOUR VISION

WAVELENGTH OF COLOUR AND COLOUR PERCEPTION

Short wavelength (approx 400–500 nm)   Violet and blue
Medium wavelength (approx 500–600 nm)   Green and yellow
Long wavelength (approx 600–700 nm)   Red

COLOUR VISION DEFECTS

Colour	Complete loss	Deficiency
Red	Protanopia ('red blindness')	Protanomaly (incomplete protanopia)
Green	Deutanopia ('green blindness')	Deutananomaly (incomplete deutanopia)
Blue	Tritanopia ('blue blindness')	Tritananomaly (incomplete tritanopia)

D15 TEST

The lines show the characteristic position of axes in various colour vision disorders (the D15 test is an adaptation of the Ishihara pseudo-isochromatic plates for graphical display of red-green defects).

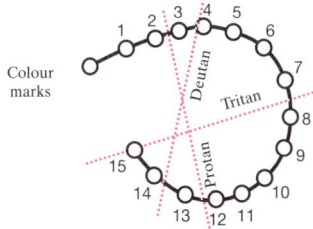

Examples of pathological findings

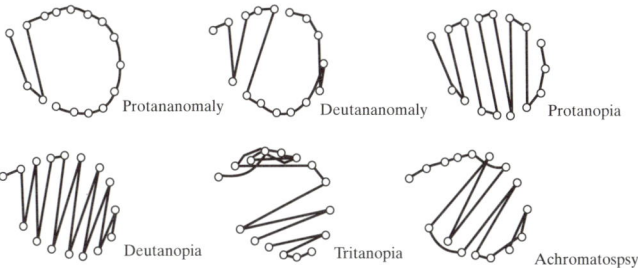

Note: The Ishihara plates (most commonly clinically used method of testing colour vision) can only identify red-green defects (most common colour defects). The American HRR plates can identify red-green and blue-yellow defects. The Fransworth Munsell 100 Hue test and anomaloscopes are more sophisticated methods of testing colour vision.

FARNSWORTH MUNSELL 100 HUE TEST

Mismatching of the colour tiles in their chromatic order is scored and then marked on a standard chart demonstrating the colour defect.

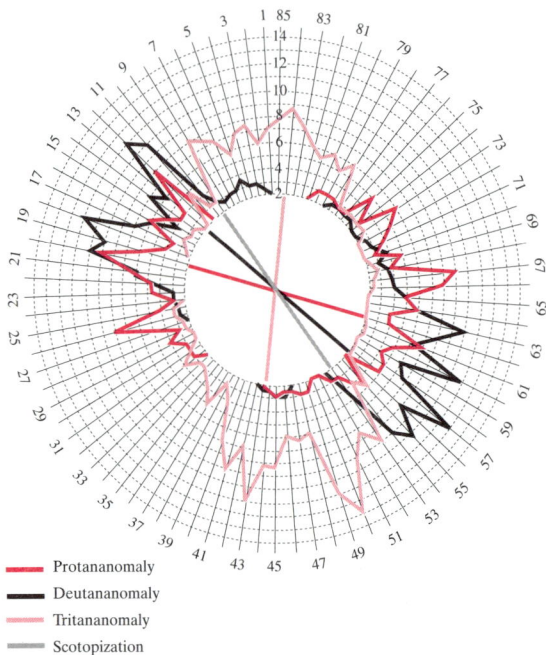

■ Protananomaly
■ Deutananomaly
■ Tritananomaly
■ Scotopization

ACQUIRED COLOUR VISION DEFECTS

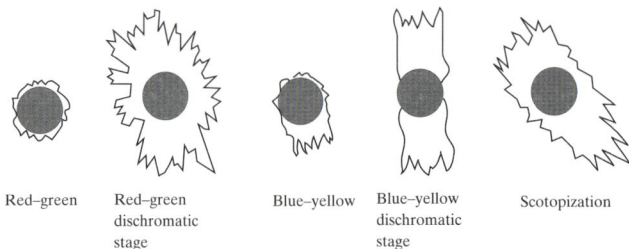

Red–green

Red–green
dischromatic
stage

Blue–yellow

Blue–yellow
dischromatic
stage

Scotopization

ANOMALOSCOPE

Upper field   Mixture of red (Li, 671 nm) and green (Hg, 546 nm)
Lower field   Yellow (Na, 589 nm)
Rayleigh's equation   Mixture equation red + green = yellow

$$\text{Anomaly ratio} \left(\text{AR}\right) = \frac{\text{red proportion of normal ratio} \times \text{green proportion of patient's setting}}{\text{green proportion of normal ratio} \times \text{red proportion of patient's setting}}$$

For example:

$$\text{Obtained ratio} = 20/15$$

$$\text{AR} = 40 \times \left(70 - 20\right)/\left(73 - 40\right) \times 20 = 3.21$$

A setting of 73 on the adjustment scale corresponds to unmixed red

Normal red–green sensitivity	AR = 1 (normal range 0.7–1.4)
Deutananomaly	AR = 2.0–20
Protananomaly	AR = 0.6–0.11
Anopia	AR not appropriate

PRINCIPLE OF EXAMINATION WITH ANOMALOSCOPE

The examined subject mixes red and green in the upper field to match the yellow in the lower field. A patient with red deficiency (protananomaly) will mix a high proportion of red, a patient with green deficiency (deutananomaly) a high proportion of green.

ANOMALOSCOPE SETTINGS WITH CORRESPONDING ANOMALY QUOTIENT (AQ)

X: patient's obtained scale adjustment, i.e. red proportion of patient's setting

X	AQ	X	AQ	X	AQ
1	87.27	25	2.33	49	0.59
2	43.03	26	2.19	50	0.56
3	28.28	27	2.07	51	0.52
4	20.91	28	1.95	52	0.59
5	16.48	29	1.84	53	0.46
6	13.54	30	1.74	54	0.43
7	11.43	31	1.64	55	0.40
8	9.85	32	1.55	56	0.37
9	8.62	33	1.47	57	0.34
10	7.64	34	1.39	58	0.31
11	6.83	35	1.32	59	0.29
12	6.16	36	1.25	60	0.26
13	5.59	37	1.18	61	0.24
14	5.11	38	1.12	62	0.22
15	4.69	39	1.06	63	0.19

X	AQ	X	AQ	X	AQ
16	4.32	40	1.00	64	0.17
17	3.99	41	0.95	65	0.15
18	3.70	42	0.89	66	0.13
19	3.44	43	0.85	67	0.11
20	3.21	44	0.80	68	0.09
21	3.00	45	0.75	69	0.07
22	2.81	46	0.71	70	0.05
23	2.64	47	0.67	71	0.03
24	2.47	48	0.63	72	0.02

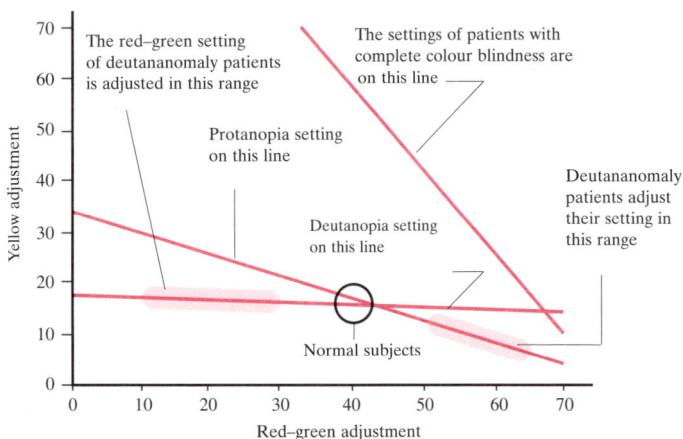

CONGENITAL COLOUR VISION DEFECTS

ACHROMATOPSIA (CONGENITAL TOTAL COLOUR BLINDNESS, ROD MONOCHROMASIA)

Physiology	Intact rods; cone dysfunction; often incomplete manifestations (residual cone function)
Symptoms	Visual acuity ~6/60; nystagmus; better vision and no nystagmus in incomplete manifestation
Diagnosis	Anomaloscope, ERG, fundoscopy (exclusion of cone dystrophy)
Inheritance	Usually autosomal recessive (both men and women can be affected)
Therapy	Red filter contact lenses are helpful

BLUE CONE MONOCHROMASIA ('ATYPICAL CONGENITAL ACHROMATOPSIA')

General	Only known cone monochromasia; blue monochromasia is easily confused with rod monochromasia; rare

Diagnosis	A congenital nystagmus resolves in the first year of life; often myopia; 2–3° eccentric fixation (usually above the foveola); confirmation of diagnosis with measurement of spectral sensitivity
Inheritance	X-linked
Therapy	Spectacles with blue lens (a visual acuity of 6/18 can be achieved in most cases)

PROTANOPIA ('RED BLINDNESS')

Physiology	Dichromasia; absence of pigment for the long wavelength range of the visible spectrum (yellow cones); red is perceived 5-fold darker than in deutanopia
Diagnosis	Anomaloscope/Ishihara plates
Inheritance	X-chromosome linked
Incidence	Approximately 1% of the male population

DEUTANOPIA ('GREEN BLINDNESS')

Physiology	Absence of the middle spectral range (due to the overlap of the sensitivity curves of the other cone types, the sensitivity loss of the affected spectral range may be minimal)
Diagnosis	Anomaloscope
Inheritance	X-chromosome linked
Incidence	Approximately 2% of the male population

TRITANOPIA ('BLUE BLINDNESS')

Physiology	Affected subjects confuse blue and green and usually also orange and pink
Inheritance	Autosomal dominant
Incidence	Congenital manifestation is very rare

ANOMALOUS TRICHROMASIA: PROTANANOMALY, DEUTANANOMALY (RED DEFICIENCY, GREEN DEFICIENCY)

Physiology	A relative colour deficiency (incomplete anopia); anomalous cone population
Diagnosis	Anomaloscope
Inheritance	X-chromosome linked
Incidence	Protananomoly and deutananomaly are seen in approximately 1% and 4% of the male population, respectively

COLOUR ASTHENOPIA (SO-CALLED COLOUR AMBLYOPIA)

Diagnosis	Increased threshold of colour differentiation (prolonged stimulus application); descriptive diagnosis; acquired colour vision defect should be excluded

ACQUIRED COLOUR VISION DEFECTS

KÖLLNER'S LAW OF ACQUIRED COLOUR VISION DYSFUNCTION

Retinal disease   **Blue colour defect**
The blue cones and the rods have similar features. The blue cones will therefore be the first cone population to be affected in dystrophic processes which initially involve the rods

Optic nerve lesion   **Red–green colour defect**
The optic nerve receives fibres mainly from the cone zone (predominance of red and green receptors). Red and green defects therefore appear early in optic neuropathies

Exceptions   Hereditary disease (e.g. Stargardt's macular dystrophy, cone dystrophy) which starts from the centre of the retina, often causes initial red colour defects; glaucoma and infantile optic atrophy cause initial blue colour defect

Lens opacities absorb short-wave light. The environment therefore appears more red–yellowish (e.g. clean curtains may appear dirty).
In **acquired macular disease**, in contrast to **optic nerve lesions**, the colour vision is not significantly affected. If a colour vision defect is present, it will be in the blue–yellow range.

COLOUR VISION DEFECTS IN OPTIC NEUROPATHIES

Lesion	Colour vision defect	Anomaloscope adjustment
Acute optic neuritis	red–green	wider than normal
Previous optic neuritis	red–green	very wide
Ethambutol intoxication	red–green	wide
Leber's optic neuropathy	red–green	very wide
Juvenile dominant optic atrophy	blue	very wide

COLOUR VISION DEFECTS IN RETINOPATHIES AND PRERETINAL DISEASES

Lesion	Colour defect	Anomaloscope setting
Cataract	blue	normal
Glaucoma	blue	wide
Age-related macular degeneration	blue	wide
Diabetic retinopathy[1]	blue, red–green	wide
Central serous retinopathy	blue, occasionally also red–green	wide
Retinal vascular occlusion	blue	wider than normal
Retinitis pigmentosa[2]	blue	usually normal

| Cone dystrophy, Stargardt's macular dystrophy[3] | red | wide |
| Re-attached retinal detachment | blue | |

[1] Blue colour defect especially after panretinal photocoagulation
[2] Blue visual field predominantly affected
[3] Progressive scotopization = symptomatic achromatopsia

OCULAR NEURORADIOLOGY

COMPUTED TOMOGRAPHY (CT)

Isodense   (equivalent to the density of the cerebral cortex)
Hyperdense   (higher density with reference to the cortex, e.g. blood, bone)
Hypodense   (high water content, e.g. oedema)

Contrast enhancement is mainly indicated for investigation of vascular, inflammatory and space-occupying lesions.
Transaxial scans are parallel to the orbital floor.
Coronal slices are perpendicular to the orbital floor.
Sagittal slices

MAGNETIC RESONANCE IMAGING (MRI)

T1-weighted sequences provide excellent anatomic detail. However, bright signal intensity of the orbital fat may obscure adjacent structures such as the optic nerve.

T2-weighted sequences provide less anatomic detail than T1-weighted images. Also, longer scan times cause further weakening of detail resolution due to patient motion artefacts. However, the bright signal intensity of the vitreous humour allows improved visualization of the inner globe.

Fat suppression techniques improve visualization of structures obscured by bright fat signal intensity in T1-weighted images.

	T1	T1 (fat-suppressed)	T2
Fat			
Vitreous			
Extraocular muscles		Contrast enhancement	
Bone			
Bone marrow			
Cerebral grey matter			
Cerebral white matter			
Liquor			
Fresh bleeding (intracellular haemoglobin)			
Vessels			

Interpretation: intermediate signal (grey) 50%, moderately hyper-intense (light grey) 30%, hyper-intense (white) 10%, moderately hypo-intense (mid-grey) 70%, hypo-intense (dark grey) 90%, no signal (black)

Contra-indications for MRI

• Pacemaker
• Metallic, ferromagnetic foreign bodies, e.g. aneurysm clips

OPTICS

VISUAL ACUITY CHART

(35 cm testing distance)

			Point	Distance equivalent
95				6/240 (0.025)
874				6/120 (0.05)
2843			26	6/60 (0.1)
638	ЕШЭ	ХОО	14	6/30 (0.2)
				6/36 (0.17)
8745	ЭШШ	ОХО	10	6/24 (0.25)
63925	ПЕЭ	ХОХ	8	6/15 (0.4)
428365	ШЕП	ОХО	6	6/12 (0.5)
374258	ЭШЭ	ХХО	5	6/9 (0.67)
937826	ШПЕ	ХОО	4	6/7.5 (0.8)
428738	ЕШП	ООХ	3	6/6 (1.0)

REFRACTIVE ERRORS

CAUSES OF AMETROPIA

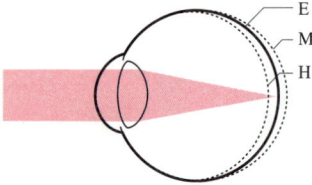

Axial ametropia

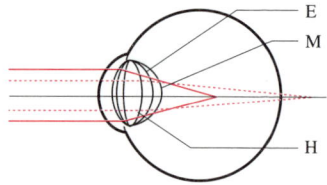

Refractive ametropia

E: Emmetropia   M: Myopia   H: Hypermetropia

Myopia
Far accommodation

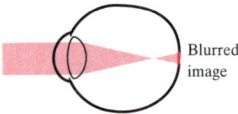

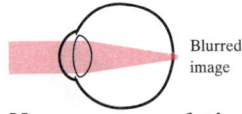

Blurred image

Near accommodation

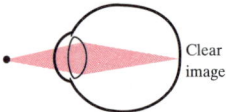

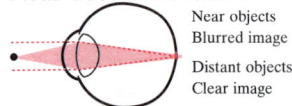

Clear image

Far accommodation with correction

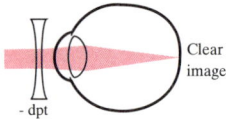

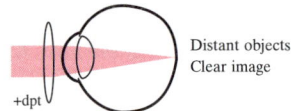

Clear image

- dpt

Hypermetropia
Far accommodation

Blurred image

Near accommodation

Near objects
Blurred image

Distant objects
Clear image

Far accommodation with correction

Distant objects
Clear image

+dpt

Near accommodation with correction

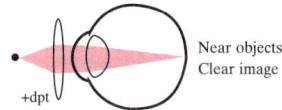

Near objects
Clear image

+dpt

ASTIGMATISM

Regular astigmatism	The principal meridians are 90° apart
Bioblique astigmatism	The principal meridians are not 90° apart
Irregular astigmatism	The principal meridians are not 90° apart and are irregular (uneven corneal surface e.g. scarring, keratoconus)
Hypermetropic astigmatism	One meridian at the plane of the retina, the other hypermetropic (behind the retina)

Myopic astigmatism	One meridian at the plane of the retina, the other myopic (in front of the retina)
Mixed astigmatism	One meridian hypermetropic, the other myopic
Composed astigmatism	Astigmatism, myopia and hypermetropia
'With the rule' astigmatism	The vertical meridian is steeper than the horizontal
'Against the rule' astigmatism	The horizontal meridian is steeper than the vertical
Oblique astigmatism	The principal meridians are at 45 ± 30° and 135 ± 30°

'With the rule' astigmatism

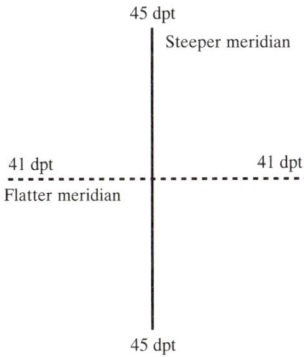

45 dpt

Steeper meridian

41 dpt — — — — — — — — — — — 41 dpt

Flatter meridian

45 dpt

'Against the rule' astigmatism

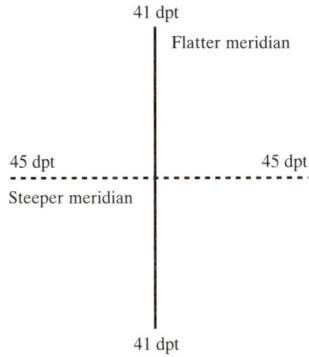

41 dpt

Flatter meridian

45 dpt — — — — — — — — — — — 45 dpt

Steeper meridian

41 dpt

CONVERSION FROM MINUS CYLINDER LENSES TO PLUS CYLINDER LENSES AND VICE VERSA

For example:

$$+2.0 \text{ sph} - 3.0 \text{ cyl}/10° \Leftrightarrow -1.0 \text{ sph} + 3.0 \text{ cyl}/100°$$

Note: the spherical equivalent (spherical value plus half of the cylinder value) does not change. In the above example: $+0.5$ sph.

CYCLOPLEGIA FOR OBJECTIVE REFRACTION

RECOMMENDED DOSAGE

Atropine

1–3 years	0.5%	1 drop every 12 hours for 2 days
	0.5%	2 drops 5 min apart, 90 min prior to planned refraction
>3 years	1%	1 drop every 12 hours for 2 days
	1%	2 drops 5 min apart, 90 min prior to planned refraction

Cyclopentolate

| <6 years | 0.5% | 3 drops 5 min apart, 20–30 min prior to planned refraction |
| >6 years | 1% | 3 drops 5 min apart, 20–30 min prior to planned refraction |

Tropicamide

| From birth onwards | 0.5% | 2 drops 5 min apart, 20 min prior to planned refraction |

OBJECTIVE REFRACTION (RETINOSCOPY)

WITH AND AGAINST MOVEMENT OF THE STREAK REFLEX

Light	Motion of streak reflex seen by examiner	Patient's far point	Correction needed
Divergent	With movement	Behind peephole of retinoscope	Add plus
	Against movement	Between patient's eye and peephole of retinoscope	Reduce plus (add minus)

FINDING NEUTRALITY AND CYLINDER AXIS

1. Fog the contralateral eye (high-power + sph).
↓

2. Adjust the distance between the filament and the convex lens of the retinoscope to allow diverging light to be emitted. Add + sph in correspondence to the 'with motion' of the streak reflex, until neutralization (patient's pupil uniformly illuminated on retinoscope flick movement) is achieved.
↓

Flick point

3. Check for astigmatism: by rotating the retinoscope sleeve, turn the streak reflex to 45° and 135°. If the streak is not in line with one of the meridians, astigmatism is present.
↓

4. Adjust sphere until streak motion achieves uniform illumination of the pupil (neutralization) in the myopic meridian and 'with movement' in the hypermetropic meridian.
↓

5. The axis of the neutralized cylinder equals the axis of the streak reflex. The axis of the other cylinder is oriented 90° away.
↓

6. Leaving the spherical lens in place, use a cylindrical lens to neutralize the second cylinder.

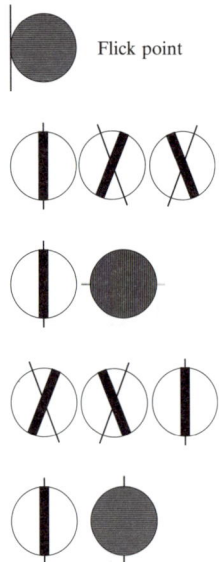

↓

7. Turn the streak reflex 90°. Confirm 'with motion' of the streak reflex. If 'with motion' does not occur, neutralization of both cylinders should be repeated.

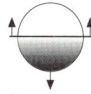

↓

8. The spherocylindrical retinoscopy can be read from the trial lens system.

↓

9. The dioptric equivalent of the examiner's working distance is subtracted from the obtained retinoscopy (e.g. subtract $+1.50$ dpt for $^2/_3$ m, $+2.00$ dpt for $^1/_2$ m).

RODENSTOCK PR 50 REFRACTOR

USING THE MANUAL RODENSTOCK PR 50 REFRACTOR

Adjust the scale to high-power +

↓

Gradually reduce + until the symbol becomes sharply focused

↓

Check for astigmatism by rotating the symbol

↓

Rotate symbol until the **uninterrupted** double line of the cross becomes sharply focused. The scale reading indicates the spherical dioptric power and the axis of the first cylinder

↓

Quickly reduce + reading until the **interrupted** double line of the cross becomes sharply focused. Record the dioptric difference from the first reading

↓

1st reading = dioptric power of sphere
Difference between 1st and 2nd readings = power of minus cylinder
Axis of 1st reading = axis of minus cylinder

MANUAL KERATOMETRY (OPHTHALMOMETRY)

Large radius (flat meridian)   ⇒   low refractive power

Small radius (steep meridian)   ⇒   high refractive power

If the astigmatism is corrected with a plus cylindrical lens, its axis is parallel to the axis of the principal meridian with the higher refractive power.

The keratometer is an instrument for measuring the central anterior corneal curvature. This is achieved by measuring the image reflected from the anterior surface of the cornea. The data are then converted into the corneal radius and the dioptric refractive power of the cornea. Only spherical values can be determined, and irregular corneal surface cannot be correctly assessed.

Newer, computer-assisted instruments for measuring corneal topography assess the entire range of the corneal curvatures (in contrast to central assessment in conventional keratometry). Irregular corneal surface such as scarring or keratoconus (irregular astigmatism) can therefore be assessed accurately.

Conventional keratometry is mainly used for assessing the corneal curvature prior to cataract surgery. In most departments manual keratometry is performed by an ophthalmic trained nurse. The illustration below shows the symbols which appear on the corneal surface using the Javal keratometer.

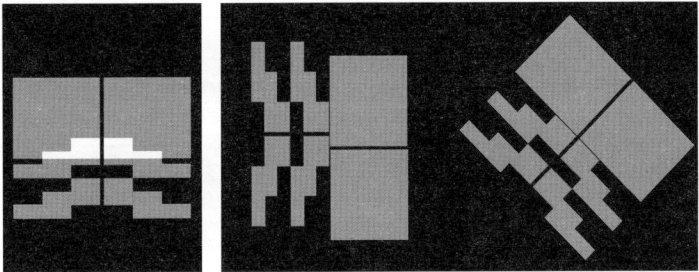

Computer-assisted corneal topography is mainly used in pre-assessment of corneal refractive surgery.

SUBJECTIVE REFRACTION

REFRACTION FOR BEST SPHERICAL CORRECTION

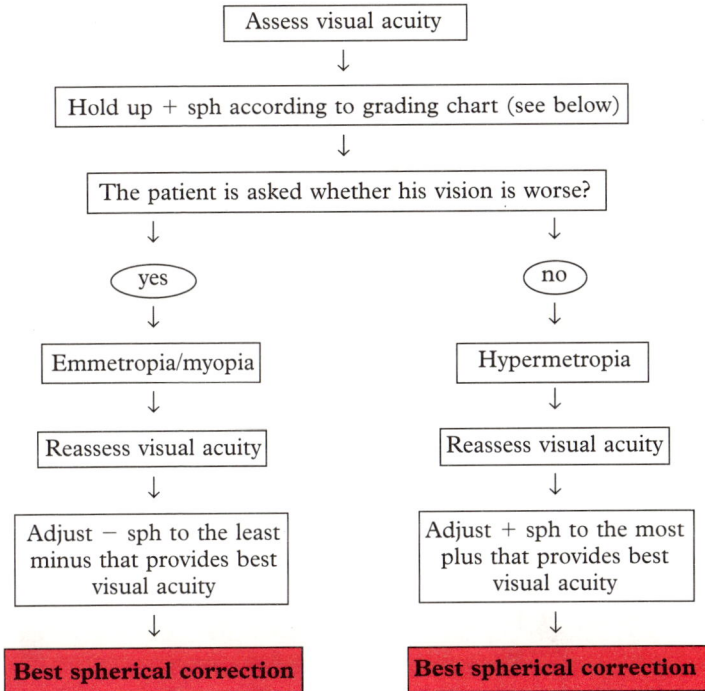

Assess visual acuity
↓

Hold up + sph according to grading chart (see below)
↓

The patient is asked whether his vision is worse?

↓   ↓

yes   no

↓   ↓

Emmetropia/myopia   Hypermetropia

↓   ↓

Reassess visual acuity   Reassess visual acuity

↓   ↓

Adjust − sph to the least   Adjust + sph to the most
minus that provides best   plus that provides best
visual acuity   visual acuity

↓   ↓

Best spherical correction   **Best spherical correction**

GRADING CHART FOR SPHERICAL LENSES

Visual acuity	Correction
<6/60	2 dpt
6/60–6/36	1 dpt
6/36–6/7.5	0.5 dpt
>6/7.5	0.25 dpt

GRADING CHART FOR TORIC LENSES

Visual acuity	Correction	Cross-cylinder
<6/60	2 dpt	±1.0 dpt
6/60–6/36	1 dpt	±0.75 dpt
6/36–6/7.5	0.5 dpt	±0.5 dpt
>6/7.5	0.25 dpt	±0.25 dpt

REFINEMENT OF CYLINDER AXIS WITH THE CROSS-CYLINDER TECHNIQUE

(cylinder power is refined after cylinder axis)

> The best subjective spherical correction and the objectively (retinoscopy) obtained cylindrical correction are placed in front of the eye

↓

> The cross-cylinder is held with its axes 45° away from the principal meridians of the positioned cylinder

↓

> The cross-cylinder is rotated back and forth and the patient asked whether positions 1 and 2 appear equal. The axis of the cylinder is recorded when the patient reports that both flip positions appear equal

REFINEMENT OF CYLINDER POWER WITH THE CROSS-CYLINDER TECHNIQUE

> The best subjective spherical correction and the cylindrical correction are placed in front of the eye (axis is refined first)

↓

> The cross-cylinder axes are held in line with the principal meridians of the positioned cylinder

↓

> Visual acuity is assessed repeatedly and the cylinder power adjusted accordingly

↓

> The spherical equivalent should remain unchanged with the sphere corrected half as much in the opposite direction as the cylinder power is altered (e.g. a 0.5 dpt cylinder power changes is accompanied by a 0.25 dpt change of sphere in the opposite direction)

NEAR CORRECTION

ESTIMATION OF THE REQUIRED NEAR CORRECTION ACCORDING TO THE PATIENT'S AGE

Age (years)	Near correction (40 cm)
45–50	0.5–1.0 dpt
50–55	1.0–2.0 dpt
>55	2.5 dpt

DETERMINING THE REQUIRED NEAR CORRECTION WITH REFERENCE TO THE RELATIVE ACCOMMODATION AMPLITUDE

Prerequisites:
• accurate distance correction
• precise working distance

↓

Place near addition (according to above table) in front of both eyes

↓

Hold near acuity chart in the patient's working distance

↓

Ask the patient to read optotypes equivalent to one grade larger than the smallest line seen with best distance correction

↓

Adjust + addition until blurring point is reached; then reduce near addition until blurring point at the other end of the amplitude is reached

↓

The best near addition equals the arithmetic mean of the values recorded at both blurring points

ACCOMMODATION AND NEAR POINT

RANGE OF ACCOMMODATION AND AGE

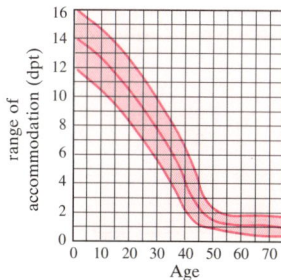

Age (years)	Range of accommodation	Near point (in emmetropia)
10	15.0 dpt	7 cm
20	10.0 dpt	10 cm
30	7.0 dpt	14 cm
40	4.5 dpt	22 cm
50	2.5 dpt	40 cm
60	1.0 dpt	100 cm
70	0.5 dpt	200 cm

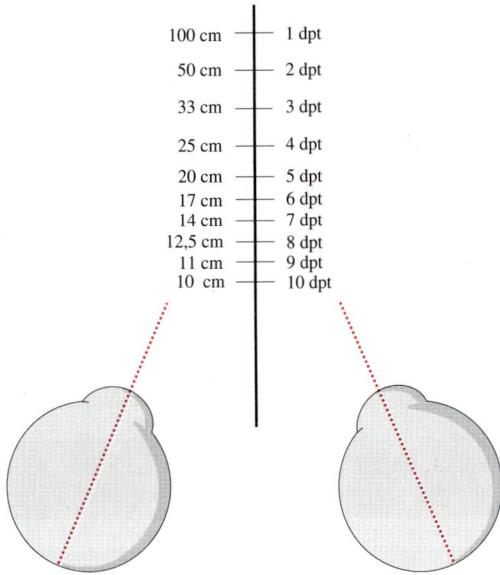

CONTACT LENS

EFFECT OF SPECTACLE LENS CORRECTION AND CONTACT LENS CORRECTION ON ACCOMMODATION EFFORT IN 33 CM DISTANCE

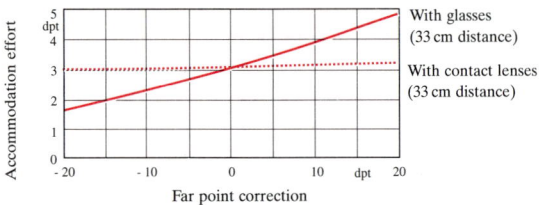

AMOUNT OF CONVERGENCE WITH SPECTACLE AND CONTACT LENS CORRECTION

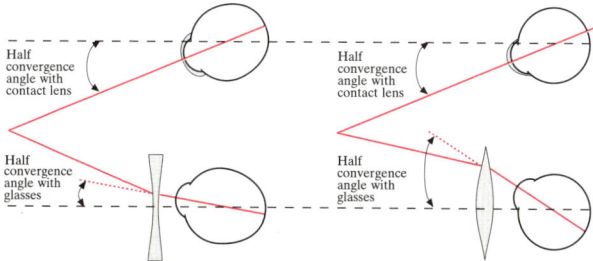

Both convergence and accommodation are increased in hypermetropic spectacle lens correction and reduced in myopic spectacle lens correction when compared with the equivalent contact lens correction.

CHANGE OF CORRECTION WHEN SWITCHING FROM SPECTACLE TO CONTACT LENS CORRECTION

Spectacle lens correction for a vertex distance of 14 mm

Hypermetropia		Myopia	
Spectacle [dpt]	Contact lens [dpt]	Spectacle [dpt]	Contact lens [dpt]
+3	+3.1	−3	−2.9
+4	+4.2	−4	−3.8
+5	+5.4	−5	−4.7
+6	+6.6	−6	−5.5
+7	+7.8	−7	−6.4
+8	+9.0	−8	−7.2
+9	+10.3	−9	−8.0
+10	+11.6	−10	−8.8
+11	+13.0	−11	−9.5
+12	+14.4	−12	−10.3
+13	+15.9	−13	−11.0
+14	+17.4	−14	−11.7
+15	+19.0	−15	−12.4

CHANGE OF RETINAL IMAGE SIZE WHEN SWITCHING FROM SPECTACLE TO CONTACT LENS CORRECTION

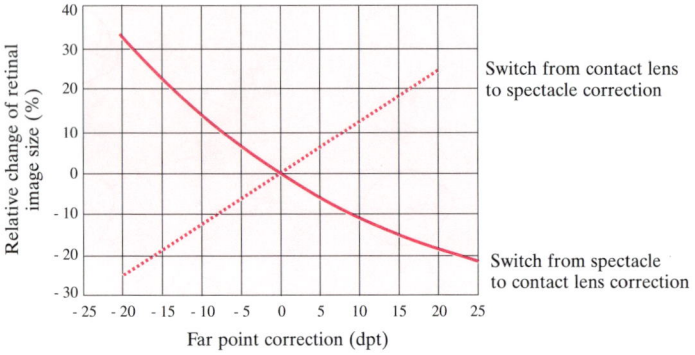

PROS AND CONS OF CONTACT LENS MATERIALS

	PMMA[a]	CAB[b]	HEMA[c]	HEMA-free	Silicon
Biological compatibility	+	+ +	−	+	+ +
Tear film function	−	(+)	+	+ +	+
Smooth surface	+	+	−	(+)	(+)
Minimal foreign body sensation	−	(−)	+ +	+ +	+
Correction of all refractive errors	+	+	−	−	−
Life span	+	(−)	−	−	−

[a] Polymethylmethacrylate
[b] Cellulose acetate butyrate
[c] Hydroxymethylacrylate

LONG-TERM COMPLICATIONS OF CONTACT LENS WEAR

• Allergic/toxic conjunctival changes
• Changes of the corneal topography
• Allergic/toxic changes of the corneal epithelium
• Trophic allergic/toxic corneal epithelial reactions
• Superficial corneal stromal reactions
• Deep stromal and endothelial changes

LENS FITTING

Total diameter of lens too small

- Increased palpebral irritation
- Increased pressure on the cornea
- Marginal reflexes
- Poor centration

Total diameter of lens too large

- Disorders of metabolism

Radius too steep

- Increased peripheral touch
- 'Spectacle blur'

Radius too flat

- Flat-fitting
- Lens liable to drop out
- Increased foreign body sensation
- Poor centration
- Unstable acuity

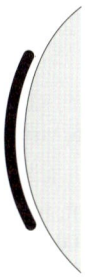

Parallel fitting   Steep fitting   Flat fitting   Cockade-shaped fitting

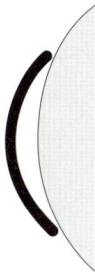

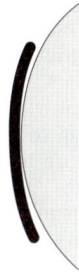

CONTACT LENS DISINFECTING SYSTEMS

Hydrogen peroxide

Disinfection with hydrogen peroxide depends on the duration the lenses are soaked in the solution. Most manufacturers recommend at least 20 minutes.

Chemical

Chemical disinfecting systems are easy to use and available for all types of soft lenses. However, soaking time is longer than with hydrogen peroxide.

Thermal

Excellent disinfection, but protein deposits remain on the lens surface and become permanently adherent. The structure of high water-content soft lenses may change.

PRE-DISINFECTION CLEANING AND POST-DISINFECTION RINSING

- Prior to disinfection, contact lenses are cleaned adequately with a surfactant, enzyme or ultrasound cleaner.
- After disinfection, a rinsing solutions is used. Rinsing solutions usually contain preservatives which may cause hypersensitivity reactions (e.g. thimerosal). Preservative-free solutions are available but are less cost-effective. Rinsing with tap water must be avoided due to the risk of acanthamoeba infection.

VISUAL AIDS

Recommendations

Visual acuity	Visual aid	Magnification in reading distance
0.2–0.4	Increased reading correction	1–2 fold
0.2–0.4	Simple magnifier	
0.1–0.3	Telescopic magnifier	2–12 fold
0.02–0.1	Screen magnifier	5–60 fold

System	Magnification	Comment
High-power near addition	Binocular up to +6.0 dpt Monocular up to +16.0 dpt	Relatively large visual field
Simple magnifier	Used for magnification of up to 4(6)-fold	Higher magnification, smaller visual field
Galilean telescope	e.g. Zeiss telescopic spectacles, 1.8-fold magnification for distance, 2–8-fold for near	Reading and television viewing for the elderly. In further deterioration, replacement of the near addition can be undertaken
Keplerian telescope	e.g. Zeiss 3.8-fold for distance, 4–8-fold for near	Advantage: longer working distance
Screen magnifier	5–60 fold (only aid to provide >8-fold magnification)	Small field

Reading a newspaper requires a visual acuity of 6/15 and a 2–4° diameter visual field.
The stronger the magnification, the smaller the visual field.
The magnification needed can be estimated by dividing 0.4 by the visual acuity with correction.
The longer the working distance of the provided system, the higher the cost.
The magnification required for a 25 cm working distance can be estimated as one quarter of the dioptric power.

Chapter 3

EYELIDS

ANATOMY OF THE EYELID

STRUCTURE OF THE UPPER LID

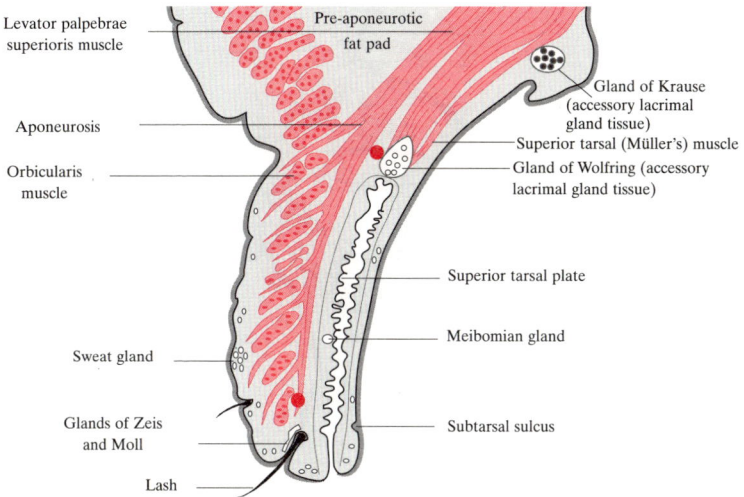

FUNCTION AND MALFUNCTION OF THE EYELID GLANDS

Name	Location	Function	Malfunction
Gland of Zeis	Hair follicles of the eyelashes on the lid margin	Sebaceous gland	External hordeolum
Gland of Moll	Hair follicles of the eyelashes on the lid margin	Sweat gland	External hordeolum
Meibomian gland	Tarsal plate	Sebaceous gland	Internal hordeolum; chalazion caused by chronic inflammation following blockage of the gland's duct

NERVE SUPPLY TO THE EYELID MUSCLES

Levator palpebrae muscle	Oculomotor nerve
Orbicularis muscle	Facial nerve

Frontalis muscle	Trigeminal nerve
Müller's muscle	Sympathetic nerves
Superior rectus muscle[1]	Oculomotor nerve
Inferior rectus muscle[1]	Ocullomotor nerve

[1] The superior rectus muscle (SRM) has connective tissue connections to the levator palpebrae muscle and there are fascial connections between the inferior rectus muscle and the lower-lid retractors (Lockwood's ligament). Hence, section of the SRM or the inferior rectus muscle (IRM) will result in lid fissure narrowing, whereas a retraction of either will lead to lid fissure widening.

BLOOD SUPPLY TO THE UPPER AND LOWER EYELIDS

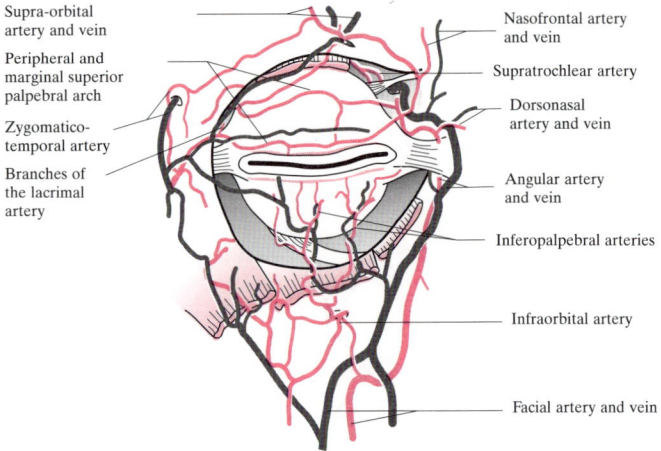

SENSORY NERVE SUPPLY TO THE UPPER AND LOWER EYELIDS

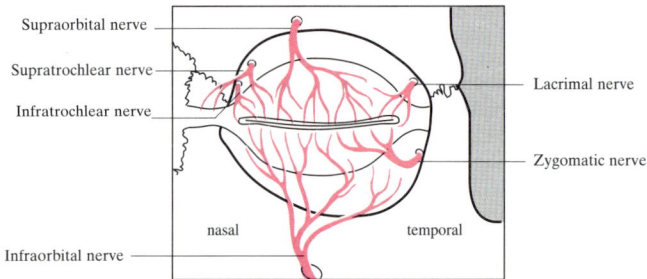

MONGOLOID AND ANTI-MONGOLOID POSITIONS OF THE EYELIDS

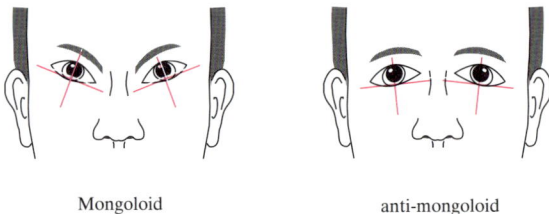

Mongoloid   anti-mongoloid

ENTROPION, ECTROPION

INVOLUTIONAL ENTROPION OF THE LOWER LID

1. Examine the lower lid in the primary position.
2. If the eyelid malposition is not manifest in the primary position, the patient is asked to look downwards and squeeze his eyelids whilst the examiner pulls the upper-lid skin outward and upward: an incipient entropion will then become obvious.
3. Evaluate the lower-lid position in the primary position and on lateral pull of the temporal canthus. Does the lower lid margin move into the normal position when under tension?
4. Test for horizontal lower lid laxity: gently pull the centre of the lower lid away from the eye and note whether the distance between the lower lid margin and the inferior limbus measures more than 5 mm.
5. Horizontal lower lid laxity is usually a bilateral condition. If not, look for cicatricial changes in the conjunctiva.
6. Examination on the slit lamp: note the position of the lower punctum and look for punctate epitheliopathy caused by trichiasis.
7. Preoperative visual acuity and photography are advisable.

Surgery: inferior retractors plication with or without lateral horizontal lid shortening; **Wies procedure; Quickert procedure**. The first requires a skin–muscle flap, the latter two a full-thickness incision.
If surgical intervention is contraindicated, everting **Quickert–Rathbun sutures** can be placed as a bedside procedure.
Note: Cicatricial conjunctival changes may require a posterior lamellar graft.

INVOLUTIONAL ECTROPION OF THE LOWER LID

1. Does the ectropion increase in up gaze?
2. Does the lower-lid margin move into the normal position on lateral pull of the temporal canthus?
3. Test for horizontal lower lid laxity as above.
4. Incomplete lid closure?
5. Cicatricial changes in the anterior tissues of the lower lid?
6. Note the position of the lower-lid punctum and check for epitheliopathy due to corneal exposure.
7. Is the lower canaliculus patent?
8. Preoperative vision and photographic record as above.

Surgery: for **horizontal lid laxity**, consider horizontal lid shortening with or without excision of excess skin (Kuhnt–Szymanowski procedure).
If the ectropion is **mainly medial without significant lid laxity**, invert the lower punctum by diamond excision of tarso-conjunctiva.
Medial ectropion with horizontal lid laxity requires Lazy-T procedure.
If the **medial canthal tendon** is lax, consider medial canthal tendon plication.
Note: Corneal exposure should be treated with lubricating agents until surgical correction is undertaken.

AESTHETIC LASER SURGERY

Blepharoplasty procedures may be combined with periocular or full-face laser-assisted skin resurfacing for cosmetic treatment of wrinkles.

Carbon dioxide (CO_2) lasers can be used for resurfacing and incisional procedures. Post-resurfacing erythema may last as long as 6 months.

Erbium: YAG energy has 13 times the affinity for water that CO_2 laser energy does. Erbium lasers, therefore, produce minimal distal thermal coagulation resulting in a quick recovery of post-operative erythema (approx. 2 weeks). Because of the minimal thermal damage, however, erbium lasers are not suitable for treatment of deep wrinkles. Neither can erbium laser be used to make incisions.

Theatre staff must be adequately trained prior to using either CO_2 or erbium lasers. Surgeons must be familiar with the Fitzpatrick classifications of skin type and with managing possible post-operative infection, scarring and pigmentary disturbances.

Laser skin resurfacing is best combined with trans-conjunctival blepharoplasty. Should, however, skin incisions be needed, conventional sutural wound closure may be replaced with cyanoacrylate tissue adhesive such as Dermabond (FDA approval expected for 1998).

PARALYTIC ECTROPION OF THE LOWER LID (SEVENTH NERVE PALSY)

1. Compare the margin reflex distance of both upper and lower lids (the distance of each upper and lower lid from the corneal light reflex allows assessment of the relative positions of all four eyelids without regard to facial asymmetry).
2. Compare the thickness of both lower-lid margins.
3. Evaluate the lid closure: check for Bell's phenomenon, measure the vertical interpalpebral distance and note possible corneal exposure.
4. Is the lower canaliculus patent?
5. Note the position of the lower punctum.
6. Preoperative vision and photographic record as above.

Surgery: lateral canthoplasty and lateral horizontal shortening (excess lower lid is resected laterally and the lateral canthal angle is then re-established using a nonabsorbable suture to secure the lower tarsal edge to the periosteum at the lateral canthus).

Cicatricial skin changes require correction with Z-plasty or replacement with a full-thickness skin graft.

Note: If spontaneous recovery occurs, treat with lubricating agents or temporary tarsorrhaphy.

PTOSIS

CAUSES OF PTOSIS

Neurogenic causes
  Oculomotor palsy
  Oculosympathetic palsy (Horner's syndrome)

Synkinetic ptosis (Marcus Gunn 'jaw-winking' syndrome)
Ophthalmoplegic migraine

Myogenic causes
Congenital:
- simple congenital ptosis
- blepharophimosis syndrome

Acquired:
- myasthenia gravis
- myasthenia-like syndromes, e.g. Eaton–Lambert syndrome
- myotonic dystrophy
- progressive external opthalmoplegia
- oculopharyngeal muscular dystrophy
- after long-term topical corticosteroid therapy

Levator aponeurosis changes
Involutional ptosis
Posttraumatic
Postsurgical stretching
Postinflammatory state
During or after pregnancy

Mechanical
External tumours of the lid, e.g. neurofibromata
Symblepharon

Pseudoptosis
Dermatochalasis
Contralateral palpebral fissure widening
Enophthalmos or contralateral exophthalmos
Duane's syndrome (palpebral fissure narrowing in adduction)
Hypertropia or contralateral hypotropia

NORMAL LID POSITION

The normal vertical diameter of the cornea is 11 mm.
In the primary position, the upper lid covers approximately 2 mm of the cornea.

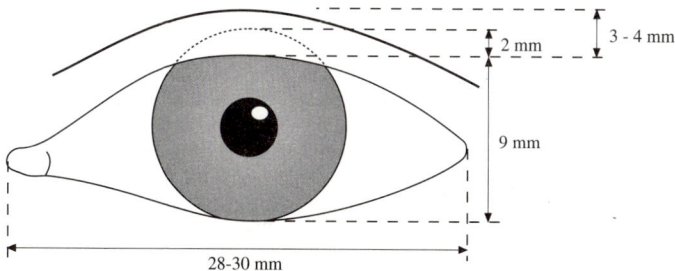

PTOSIS: ASSESSMENT

WORK-UP OF THE PTOSIS PATIENT

History
    Congenital – acquired
    Sporadic – hereditary
    Traumatic – nontraumatic
    Gradual – sudden
    Isolated – associated
    Stable – progressive

Examination
    Quantitative evaluation:
    Levator function, palpebral fissure, amount of ptosis (margin reflex distance), lid lag, position of lid skin crease

    Qualitative evaluation:
    Lid closure, Bell's phenomenon, lid movement, synkinesis e.g jaw-winking, sustained up-gaze manoeuvre, brow position, lid contour, prolapsed orbital fat, epicanthus, morphological changes (e.g. scarring, skin tumours)

Additional ophthalmic data
    Orthoptic examination, frontalis muscle function, tear production, tear film stability, pupillary reactions, biomicroscopy, fundoscopy, visual fields, electophysiology (ERG), phenylephrine 10% test.

Additional nonophthalmic data
    Refer for medical or neurological assessment if indicated (e.g. myasthenia gravis)

EVALUATION OF THE LEVATOR FUNCTION

Upper lid excursion	Levator function
Less than 2 mm	None
2–4 mm	Poor
5–7 mm	Moderate
8–15 mm	Good

Note: Maximum excursion of the lid between up-gaze and down-gaze should be measured, but the frontalis muscle must be prevented from concomitant pulling: fix the eyebrow with the thumb.

SURGERY

Levator aponeurosis tightening is indicated in ptosis with levator function of ≥11 mm. It is preferred to the Fasanella–Servat procedure, as it preserves tarsus and conjunctiva and allows re-establishment of the lid crease.
Müller's muscle resection, although (similarly to the Fasanella–Servat procedure) requiring an internal approach, should be considered in cases with good levator function and a positive phenylephrine test.
Levator resection is indicated in cases with moderate levator function (5–10 mm).

Frontalis suspension procedures are performed in patients with poor levator function (less than 5 mm). In Marcus Gunn jaw-winking syndrome, frontalis suspension to both upper lids is recommended to avoid asymmetry in down-gaze.

Brow elevation as a primary procedure or as an adjunct should always be considered in the presence of brow ptosis.

PTOSIS: CONGENITAL PTOSIS

EVALUATION OF CONGENITAL PTOSIS

[Beard C (1976) Ptosis, 2nd edn, Mosby, St Louis]

Amount of ptosis	Degree of ptosis
2 mm	Mild
3 mm	Moderate
4 mm and over	Severe

PREOPERATIVE EVALUATION FOR CONGENITAL PTOSIS CORRECTION

[Beard C (1976) Ptosis, 2nd edn, Mosby, St Louis]

Levator function	Amount of ptosis	Extent of resection
8 mm or more	2 mm	10–13 mm
	3 mm	14–17 mm
5–7 mm	2 mm	14–17 mm
	3 mm	18–22 mm
	4 mm	23 mm or more with excision of any excess skin
2–4 mm	3 mm	18–22 mm
	4 mm	23 mm or more with excision of any excess skin

DOCUMENTATION OF EXAMINATION DATA IN THE PTOSIS PATIENT

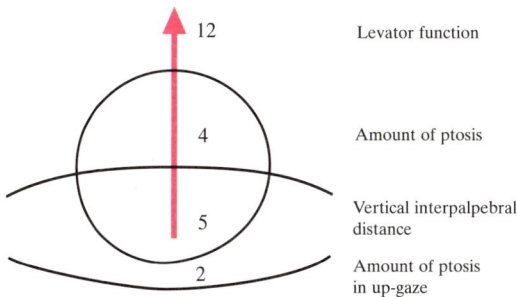

12	Levator function
4	Amount of ptosis
5	Vertical interpalpebral distance
2	Amount of ptosis in up-gaze

Note: The amount of ptosis is the difference between the measured and the normal amount of uncovered cornea. For example, if the vertical line of uncovered cornea in the primary position measures 5 mm (normally it measures 9 mm, as the upper lid covers 2 mm below the superior limbus), then the amount of ptosis is 4 mm.

RELEVANT DATA FOR DIFFERENTIAL DIAGNOSIS IN THE PTOSIS PATIENT

Vertical interpalpebral distance in down-gaze	The normal lid fissure widening in down-gaze usually measures 2–3 mm, whereas it measures more than 3 mm in **congenital ptosis** (lid lag)
Position of the eyebrow	The eyebrow is normally positioned directly in front of the supraorbital ridge, whereas it is in a lower position in brow ptosis (**brow droop**)
Position of the lid skin crease	The lid crease is normally positioned 5–8 mm above the upper lid margin. Involutional ptosis shows a high lid crease
Synkinesis?	**Marcus Gunn 'jaw-winking' syndrome** is characterized by momentary lid retraction of the ptotic eye on opening the mouth or moving the jaw. Marcus Gunn ptosis is usually unilateral and may be associated with superior rectus weakness **Aberrant regeneration of third nerve palsy** shows bizarre upper lid motility such as elevation on attempted adduction or down-gaze
Sustained up-gaze manoeuvre	Fatigue of the upper lid after 30 seconds up-gaze indicates **myasthenia gravis**
Anisocoria?	**Horner's syndrome** presents with 1–2 mm ptosis and ipsilateral miosis (poor pupillary dilation to cocaine confirms the diagnosis)

CONGENITAL PTOSIS VERSUS ACQUIRED PTOSIS

	Congenital	Acquired
Incidence	65–90%	Rare
History	Ask for early childhood photographs (nonprogressive)	Gradual or sudden presentation, again ask or compare with previous photographs
Signs	Lid lag; lateral S-shaped upper lid in congenital myogenic ptosis	No lid lag
Postoperative result	Undercorrection more likely; rarely remaining overcorrection	High risk of over-correction

ESSENTIAL BLEPHAROSPASM

Essential blepharospasm

Definition	Involuntary, tonic, bilateral contraction of the orbicularis oculi, procerus and corrugator muscles
Onset	Usually not before 50 years of age

Sex ratio	Female : male 3 : 1
Aetiology	Unknown
Course	Insidious beginning, which over months or years progresses to forceful uninterrupted eyelid spasm causing severe visual disability
Involvement of the lower facial muscle	If the blepharospasm extends to other facial muscles, it is referred to as Meige's syndrome (idiopathic orofacial dystonia) or Brueghel's syndrome (idiopathic oromandibular dystonia); the latter named after the distorted facial expression of a subject in a Brueghel painting
Differential diagnosis	Reflex blepharospasm due to photophobia or irritation as in keratitis or uveitis, eyelid myokymia, tics and habit spasms, hemifacial spasm[1], apraxia of eyelid opening, drug-induced blepharospasm (tardive dyskinesia), Parkinson's
Work-up	History, drug history, ophthalmic and neurological examination, imaging of the brain and posterior fossa to exclude compressing lesions
Medical treatment	Psychotherapy is of debatable value; lorazepham, clonazepam and muscle relaxants may be of some use, but recently botulinum A toxin injections have become the treatment of first choice, in which onset of symptomatic relief occurs two to three days after injection and lasts for three months. Main side-effects (ptosis, sicca syndrome, diplopia, ectropion) can be avoided by sparing the central parts of the upper lids and the central and medial parts of the lower lids
Surgical treatment	Surgical intervention includes resection of the temporal and zygomatic branches of the facial nerve or subtotal removal of the eyelid protractors. The latter is associated with fewer side-effects than the first, but both procedures are indicated only in cases of failure of previous medical treatment.

[1] Hemifacial spasm usually respects the midline, but it may occasionally be bilateral, successfully mimicking essential blepharospasm. Note, though, that in the first the spasm remains during sleep, whereas in the latter it usually resolves with sleep or under general anaesthesia.

SYNOPSIS OF EYELID LESIONS

BENIGN AND MALIGNANT EYELID LESIONS

Lesion	Characteristics	Pathology
Benign lesions		
Xanthelasma	Usually bilateral; yellowish; well defined	Subcutaneous lipoprotein deposits
Papilloma	Very common; broad-based or pedunculated	Irregular, elevated skin proliferation

Pigmented naevus	Present at birth with later pigmentation	Rarely becomes malignant
Molluscum contagiosum	Multiple small nodules with central depression	Virus infection
Milia	Multiple small, pale, superficial lesions without central depression	Small epidermal inclusion cysts
Cyst	Gland of Moll; gland of Zeis; sebaceous gland	Cyst formation due to blockage of the gland's duct
Dermoid	Firm subcutaneous mass most common along the superotemporal orbital rim	Choristoma
Actinic keratosis	Potential for malignant transformation into a squamous cell carcinoma; occurs in fair-skinned people on areas of skin exposed to sun	Hyperkeratosis
Cutaneous horn	May be associated with actinic keratosis	Hyperkeratosis
Neurofibroma	Frequently widely distributed over the body; associated with café-au-lait spots	Phacomatosis
Capillary haemangioma	Presentation usually in the first months after birth	Hamartoma
Cavernous haemangioma	Most common benign tumour of orbit among adults	Hamartoma
Lymphangioma	Uncommon; often enlarges because of internal haemorrhage ('chocolate cysts')	Hamartoma
Naevus flammeus	May be associated with cerebral angioma and glaucoma (Sturge–Weber syndrome)	Phacomatosis

Malignant lesions

Basal cell carcinoma	Most common malignant tumour of the eyelid; often localized on sun-exposed lower lids and lower medial canthal areas	Nodular, ulcerative and sclerosing types, the latter particularly likely to be infiltrative
Squamous cell carcinoma	Usually in older patients; potential metastasis to regional lymph nodes	Marked cellular atypia; dyskeratosis; loss of the epidermis

Sebaceous gland carcinoma	Highly malignant; may mimic chalazions	Multifocal occurrence possible
Malignant melanoma	Strongly dark brown pigmentation	Loss of normal polarity; invasion of the epithelium followed by invasion of the dermis; atypical cells
Kaposi's sarcoma	Frequently associated with AIDS	Many foci of capillary clusters in a stroma of malignant spindle cells

Chapter 4

CONJUNCTIVA/LACRIMAL SYSTEM

ANATOMY OF THE LACRIMAL SYSTEM

LACRIMAL SYSTEM

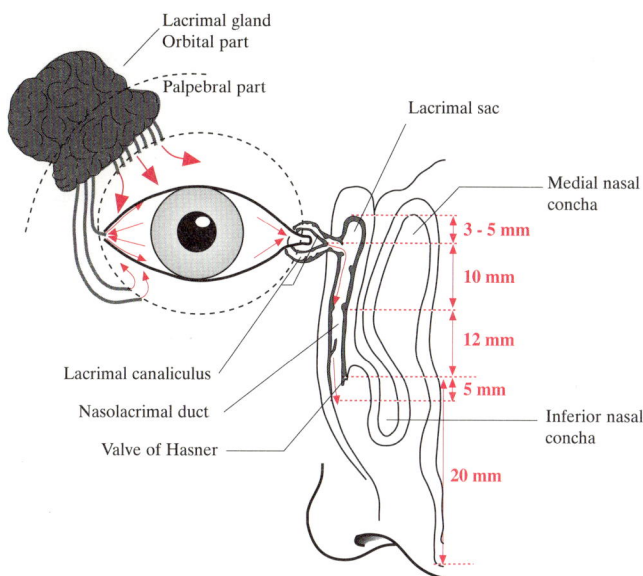

NERVE SUPPLY OF THE LACRIMAL GLAND

Lacrimal nerve	Secretion
Sympathetic fibres	Sympathetic
Abducens	Sensory

COMPOSITION OF THE TEAR FILM

THE GLANDS THAT TAKE PART IN THE PRODUCTION OF THE PRE-CORNEAL TEAR FILM

Lipid secretions

Meibomian glands	In the tarsal plate
Glands of Zeis	Ciliary follicles

Aqueous secretions

Glands of Krause	Palpebral conjunctiva
Glands of Wolfring	Palpebral conjunctiva
Glands of Moll	Ciliary follicles
Lacrimal gland	Anterotemporal part of the orbital roof with approximately 10 ducts in the superolateral fornix and in the superior palpebral conjunctiva

Mucin secretions

Goblet cells	Bulbar and tarsal conjunctiva
Crypts of Henle	Palpebral conjunctiva
Glands of Manz	Limbal conjunctiva (round the cornea)

TEAR FILM COMPOSITION

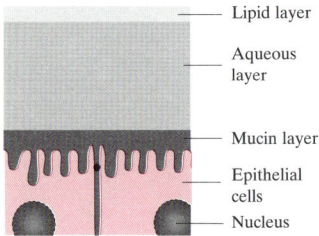

- Lipid layer
- Aqueous layer
- Mucin layer
- Epithelial cells
- Nucleus

LOCATION OF GLANDS

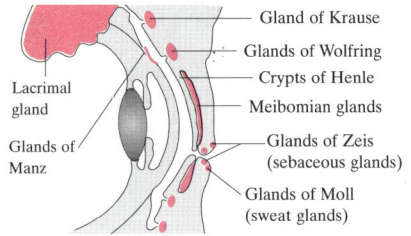

- Gland of Krause
- Glands of Wolfring
- Crypts of Henle
- Meibomian glands
- Glands of Zeis (sebaceous glands)
- Glands of Moll (sweat glands)

Lacrimal gland
Glands of Manz

THE TEAR FILM LAYERS AND THEIR FUNCTIONS

Layer; thickness	Function
Superficial lipid layer; ~0.1 μm	Inhibition of evaporation of the underlying watery layer, surface tension
Middle aqueous layer; 6–9 μm	Epithelial metabolism, defence against invading organisms
Inner mucin layer; less than 0.1 μm	Enables wetting of the hydrophobic epithelium by the aqueous layer

SPECIAL TESTS FOR EVALUATION OF TEAR FILM DISORDERS

SCHIRMER I TEST

Materials	Standardized (Whatman) filter paper (5 × 35 mm)
Method	No anaesthesia Filter paper is placed in the temporal third of the lower lid Patient is asked to keep the eyes in slight supraduction Filter paper removed after 5 min
Interpretation	10–30 mm is considered normal

BASIC SECRETION TEST

Materials	Standardized (Whatman) filter paper (5 × 35 mm) Topical anaesthetic
Method	Instillation of topical anaesthesia Lower fornix is dried gently Filter paper is placed in the temporal third of the lower lid Patient is asked to keep the eyes in slight supraduction Filter paper removed after 5 min
Interpretation	10–15 mm is considered normal

SCHIRMER II TEST

Materials	Standardized (Whatman) filter paper (5 × 35 mm) Topical anaesthetic Cotton wool applicator
Method	Instillation of topical anaesthesia Lower fornix is dried gently Filter paper is placed in the temporal third of the lower lid Patient is asked to keep the eyes in slight supraduction Irritation of the nasal mucosa with a cotton wool applicator Filter paper removed after 2 min
Interpretation	>15 mm is considered normal

TEAR FILM BREAK-UP TIME

Materials	Fluorescein dye or fluorescein strip Slit lamp with cobalt blue filter

Method	No anaesthesia
	Installation of fluorescein dye into the lower fornix
	Patient is asked to blink several times
	Time is measured between last blink and the appearance
	    of the first dry spot indicating a break-up of the
	    otherwise uniform tear film
	The average of three consecutive measurements is
	    documented

Interpretation	>10 sec is considered normal

ROSE BENGAL STAINING

Materials	Rose Bengal dye
Method	No anaesthesia Installation of a small drop of rose bengal dye into the lower fornix

Disadvantage	Marked ocular irritation (topical anaesthesia may cause a false positive result)
Interpretation	Mild dry eye: pink staining of nasal and temporal conjunctiva
	Filamentary keratitis: pink stained dead and devitalized epithelial cells and mucus on the corneal surface

Note: Rose Bengal dye is superior to fluorescein dye in demonstrating early keratoconjunctivitis sicca.

CAUSES OF DRY EYE

AQUEOUS TEAR LAYER

Hyposecretion of the lacrimal gland

Congenital

Lacrimal gland aplasia (congenital alacrima)
Lacrimal gland hypoplasia (Bonnevie Ullrich syndrome)
Anhydrotic ectodermal dysplasia
Neurogenic hyposecretion
Aplasia of lacrimal nerve nucleus
Familial dysautonomia (Riley–Day syndrome)
Cystic fibrosis

Acquired

Senile atrophy of the lacrimal gland
Traumatic, inflammatory or neoplastic disease of the lacrimal gland
Hypofunction of the lacrimal gland associated with systemic disease:
  Sjögren's syndrome, rheumatoid arthritis, benign lymphomyoepithelial lesion of the parotid gland (Godwin), sarcoidosis, psoriasis arthropathica, lupus erythematosus, scleroderma, periarteritis nodosa, amyloidosis, leukaemic infiltration, acquired immune deficiency syndrome (AIDS), graft versus host disease
Neurogenic hyposecretion
  Facial nerve lesion, greater superficial petrosal nerve lesion, pterygopalatine ganglion lesion, lesion of the communicating branch of the lacrimal nerve
Toxic hyposecretion
  Atropine, botulinum, beta-blockers
Psychogenic hypolacrima

Increased tear film evaporation

Exophthalmos, lagophthalmos, ectropion, insufficient lid closure, blink reflex malfunction (Vth cranial), environmental factors

LIPID LAYER

Chronic blepharitis, acne rosacea

MUCIN LAYER

Vitamin A deficiency
Peri-menopause
Ocular pemphigoid
Infectious diseases
   Diphtheria, trachoma, Reiter's syndrome, smallpox, acute (epidemic)
   keratoconjunctivitis
Dermatological diseases
   Erythema multiforme (Stevens–Johnson syndrome), pemphigoid vulgaris,
   dermatitis herpetiformis, epidermolysis bullosa, ichthyosiform
   erythroderma, exfoliative dermatitis, ichthyosis congenita

ABNORMAL CORNEAL EPITHELIUM (MICROVILLI LOSS)

INFLAMMATION OF THE LACRIMAL SYSTEM

ACUTE DACRYOCYSTITIS VERSUS CHRONIC DACRYOCYSTITIS

	Acute	Chronic
Symptoms	Pain	Epiphora
	Redness	Mucopurulent discharge
	Swelling	
	Epiphora	
	Purulent discharge	
Investigations	Microbiology	Microbiology
	ENT referral	ENT referral
Treatment	Local and systemic antibiotics	Dacryocystectomy
	Warm compresses	Dacryocystorhinostomy
	Incision?	

CAUSES OF SWELLING OF THE LACRIMAL GLAND

Acute

Infection   Bacterial: staphylococci, streptococci, *Haemophilus influenzae*
          (children)
        Viral: mumps, Epstein–Barr virus, herpes viruses, cytomegalovirus
        Fungal

Chronic

Infection	Tuberculosis, syphilis
Systemic disease	Sjögren's syndrome, sarcoidosis
Tumour	Adenocystic carcinoma, lymphoma

MELANOCYTIC CONJUNCTIVAL LESIONS/LYMPHATIC DRAINAGE OF THE EYELIDS AND CONJUNCTIVA

CLASSIFICATION OF PIGMENTARY CHANGES OF THE CONJUNCTIVA

I.   **Epithelial melanosis**

II. **Naevi**
     Junctional
     Subepithelial
     Compound

III. **Congenital melanosis of oculi**
     Blue naevus
     Naevus of Ota
     Oculodermal melanocytosis

IV. **Acquired melanosis**
     Primary acquired melanosis
     Secondary acquired melanosis

V.   **Malignant melanoma**

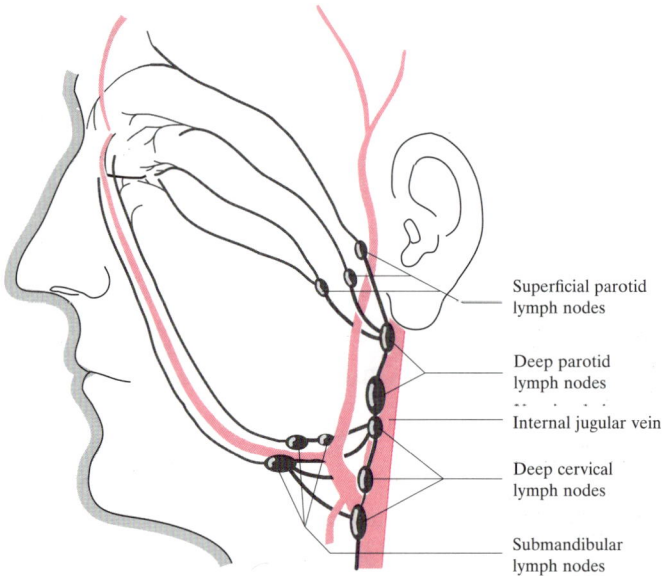

Superficial parotid lymph nodes

Deep parotid lymph nodes

Internal jugular vein

Deep cervical lymph nodes

Submandibular lymph nodes

CONJUNCTIVITIS

CONJUNCTIVAL (SUPERFICIAL) INJECTION VERSUS CILIARY (DEEP) INJECTION

	Conjunctival injection	Ciliary injection
Cause	Conjunctivitis	Keratitis, uveitis (iritis)
Colour	Red	Dark red
Location	Mainly peripheral, less pronounced near the limbus	Subconjunctival, pericorneal
Affected vessels	Superficial vessels; move with the conjunctiva; can be blanched with 1 : 1000 adrenaline or 10% phenylephrine	Deep vessels; do not move with the conjunctiva; can not be blanched with topical vasoconstrictive agents. Also scleritis/episcleritis

SYMPTOM MANIFESTATION IN VIRAL, BACTERIAL, CHLAMYDIAL AND ALLERGIC CONJUNCTIVITIDES

	Viral	Bacterial	Chlamydial	Allergic
Acute	+	+	+	+
Irritation	−	−	−	++
Hyperaemia	+	++	+	+
Haemorrhages	±	±	−	−
Chemosis	±			++
Epiphora	++	+	+	+
Discharge	+, watery	++, purulent	mucopurulent	±, mucoid
Pseudo-membranes	±	±	−	−
Papillae	−	+	±	+
Follicles	+	−	++	−
Pre-auricular lymph node swelling	+	±	+	−
Pannus	−	−	+	−
Keratitis	±	±	+	−
Upper respiratory tract infection, fever	±	±	−	−
Cytology	Lymphocytes, monocytes	Granulocytes, bacteria	Cytoplasmic inclusion bodies, leukocytes, plasma cells	Eosinophil granulocytes, lymphocytes

++ marked; + moderate; ± occasionally; − rarely.

NEONATAL CONJUNCTIVITIS

Aetiology	Manifestation	Symptoms	Microbiology
Chemical (silver nitrate, antibiotics)	Several hours after birth	Hyperaemia, some mucoid discharge	–
Gonococcal	2–4 days after birth	Acute purulent conjunctivitis	Intracellular Gram-negative diplococci; culture on chocolate agar or Thayer–Martin for *Neisseria gonorrhoea* and culture on blood agar for other bacteria
Other bacteria	3–20 days after birth	Mucopurulent conjunctivitis	Gram-positive or Gram-negative bacteria; blood agar culture media
Chlamydial	5–12 days after birth	Mucopurulent (rarely purulent) conjunctivitis	Cytoplasmic inclusion bodies
Herpetic	1–3 weeks after birth	Blepharo-conjunctivitis, corneal ulcers, systemic disease	Polynuclear giant cells, intranuclear inclusion bodies

DIFFERENTIAL DIAGNOSIS OF BACTERIAL CONJUNCTIVIDES

Organism	Discharge	Irritation	Location	Corneal involvement	Pre-auricular lymph node swelling	Gram staining
Staphylococcus	muco-purulent	moderate	generalized	epithelial keratopathy	rare	positive
Haemophilus	muco-purulent	moderate	generalized	rare	common	negative
Pneumococcus	purulent	–	generalized	ulceration	rare	positive
Moraxella	minimal	moderate	corners of lid fissure	ulceration	rare	negative
Pseudomonas	purlulent	–	generalized	ulceration (common)	rare	negative
Gonococcus	muco-purulent	–	generalized, unilateral in adults	ulceration	rare	negative

BACTERIAL CONJUNCTIVITIS

GRAM STAINS OF THE MOST IMPORTANT ORGANISMS CAUSING BACTERIAL CONJUNCTIVITIS

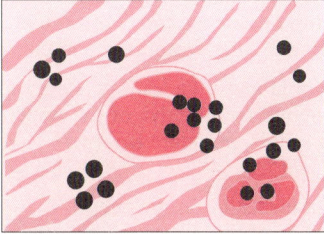

Staphylococci:
Gram-positive

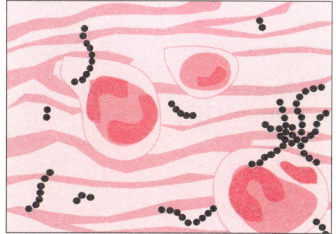

Streptococci:
Gram-positive

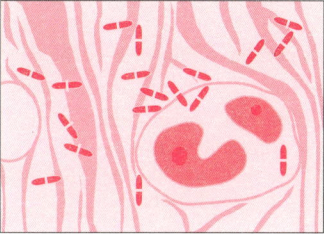

Moraxella lacunata:

Gram-negative double rods

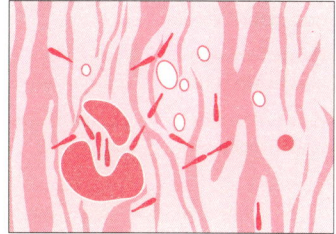

Haemophilus aegypticus
(Koch–Weeks):
Gram-negative rods

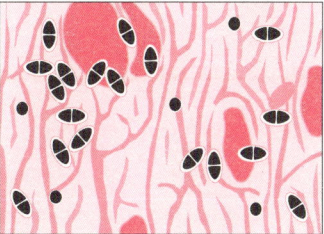

Pneumococci:
Gram-positive diplococci

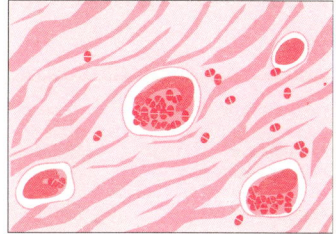

Gonococci:
Intracellular Gram-negative
diplococci

Conjunctivitis	Organism	Typical features
Staphylococcal conjunctivitis	*Staphylococcus aureus*	Usually subacute or chronic infection, purulent discharge, variable picture
Pneumococcal conjunctivitis	*Streptococcus pneumoniae*	Acute purulent infection, chemosis, multiple subconjunctival haemorrhages
Haemophilus conjunctivitis	*Haemophilus influenzae*	Sub-acute or chronic infection, often with pre-auricular lymph node swelling
Inclusion conjunctivitis	*Chlamydia trachomatis* (serotypes D–K)	Hyperaemia and follicles (late stage) in the palpebral conjunctiva of the upper and lower lids, punctate keratitis (upper half)
Trachoma	*Chlamydia trachomatis* (serotypes A–C)	Lymph follicles in the palpebral conjunctiva of the upper lid, cicatricial entropion, trichiasis, corneal scarring
Gonococcal conjunctivitis	*Neisseria gonorrhoea*	Acute purulent conjunctivitis, corneal ulceration
Angular blepharo-conjunctivitis	*Moraxella lacunata*	Subacute infection of the lid fissure corners and the adjacent lid margins
Pseudomonas conjunctivitis	*Pseudomonas aeruginosa*	Purulent conjunctivitis with corneal ulceration
Koch–Weeks conjunctivitis	*Haemophilus aegypticus*	Highly infectious conjunctivitis with chemosis, subconjunctival haemorrhages, lid swelling and corneal ulceration; warm climate
Diphtheria conjunctivitis	*Corynebacterium diphtheriae*	Lid oedema, conjunctival necrosis, pseudomembranes
Tubercular conjunctivitis	*Mycobacterium tuberculosis*	Chronic granulomatous conjunctivitis

FOLLICULAR CONJUNCTIVITIS

Organism or disease	Discharge	Conjunctival changes	Corneal involvement	Microbiology	Aetiology and duration
Molluscum contagiosum	Watery	Follicles, papillae	Superficial epithelial keratopathy, pannus	Monocytes, molluscum inclusion bodies in the biopsy	Molluscum virus, chronic (quick recovery usually achieved with excision)

Organism or disease	Discharge	Conjunctival changes	Corneal involvement	Microbiology	Aetiology and duration
Adult inclusion conjunctivitis	Muco-purulent	Tarsal follicles and papillae	Epithelial keratopathy, micropannus, sub-epithelial infiltrates	Leukocytes, monocytes, cytoplasmic inclusion bodies	*Chlamydia trachomatis*, chronic (3–5 months)
Trachoma	Muco-purulent	Follicles on the upper tarsus, papillae, conjunctival scarring	Superficial punctate keratitis, prominent pannus	Leukocytes, monocytes, plasma cells, inclusion bodies	*Chlamydia trachomatis*, chronic (years)
Moraxella	Little	Angular conjunctivitis, tarsal follicles	Marginal infiltrates	Gram-negative diplobacilli, leukocytes	*Moraxella lacunata*, chronic
Masquerade conjunctivitis	Mucoid	Follicles with phagocytosed pigment	None	Pigmented granula	Cosmetics, adrenaline
Axenfeld's follicular conjunctivitis	Little	Follicles on the lower tarsus	None	Monocytes	Viral, 1–2 years
Thygeson's conjunctivitis	Little	Follicles on the palpebral conjunctiva (lower fornix)	Superficial epithelial keratopathy	Leukocytes	Unknown, 5 months
Drug-induced conjunctivitis	Variable	Follicles, scarring, dry eye	Keratitis, pseudo-dendrites, pannus, limbal follicles	Lymphocytes, leukocytes	Idoxuridine, atropine, antibiotics

CHLAMYDIAL CONJUNCTIVITIS

MACCALLAN'S CLASSIFICATION OF TRACHOMA

[MacCallan AF (1931) Epidemiology in trachoma. *Br J Ophthalmol* **15**:389–511]

Stage	Clinical features
I (early)	Nonspecific conjunctival irritation, immature follicles on the palpebral conjunctiva
II (manifest)	Lymph follicles on the upper tarsal plate, typical superficial corneal vascularization (pannus trachomatosus)
III (scarring)	Follicles become necrotic and conjunctival scarring begins to form (limbal Herbert's pits, von Arlt's lines on the superior tarsus)
IV (complicated)	Cicatricial entropion, trichiasis, corneal ulceration and scarring

WHO GRADING OF TRACHOMA

[Dawson CR, Jones BB, Tarizzo ML (1981) Guide to Trachoma Control in Programmes for Prevention of Blindness. WHO, Geneva]

Grade	Papillary reaction	Follicular reaction
I (bland)	0–2	0–1
II (mild)	0–2	2
III (moderate)	1–2	3
IV (severe)	3	0–3 (follicles may be obscured by papillae)

TRACHOMA VERSUS PARATRACHOMA

	Trachoma	Paratrachoma
Organism	*Chlamydia trachomatis* (serotypes A–C)	*Chlamydia trachomatis* (serotypes D–K)
Transmission	Ocular	Oculogenital
Epidemiology	Endemic, hyperendemic	Sporadic
Incubation period	5–8 days	8–10 days; occasionally only 6 days in infants
Endemic region	Developing countries	Industrialized countries
Ocular involvement	Bilateral	Unilateral, bilateral
Initial manifestation	Conjunctival follicles	Conjunctival follicles
Complications	Corneal involvement, cicatricial entropion, trichiasis	None
Course	Chronic (years)	Weeks
Therapy	Topical and oral tetracycline or erythromycin	Topical and oral tetracycline or erythromycin
Prognosis	Poor in chronic cases with continuous re-infection	Good

Chapter 5

CORNEA/SCLERA

ANATOMY OF THE CORNEA

THE CORNEAL LAYERS

Layer	Features	Function
Epithelium	Thickness of ~0.05 mm, thicker peripherally (up to 10 layers of cells) and thinner centrally (5–6 layers of cells); the superficial cells are flat and show microvilli on their outer surface; the basal columnar cells are attached to the basal membrane with hemi-desmosomes; regeneration occurs about once weekly	Barrier to hydrophilic materials; microvilli and microplicae extend into the mucin layer of the tear film. Maintaining a smooth optical border surface for light refraction
Bowman's membrane	Acellular collagen fibre membrane; its inner surface merges into the substantia propria	No posttraumatic regeneration; defects cause scar formation. Mechanical protection of stroma
Stroma (substantia propria)	90% of the corneal thickness; multiple lamellae of collagen fibres that run parallel to the corneal surface and parallel to each other in the same lamella but at right angles to the next lamella	The regular structure of the avascular stroma and its low water content produce high corneal transparency. Elasticity and stability
Descemet's membrane	The basement membrane of the endothelium; increased thickness with age	Injury causes retraction and separation from the stroma
Endothelium	A single layer of polygonal cells; permeability depends on molecular size. Critical cellular density of <500–1000 cells per mm^2. Danger of bullous keratopathy (caused by pump failure)	No posttraumatic regeneration; defects cause migration and enlargement of adjacent cells; endothelial pump failure leads to corneal oedema. Stroma dehydration to maintain transparency. Diffusion barrier

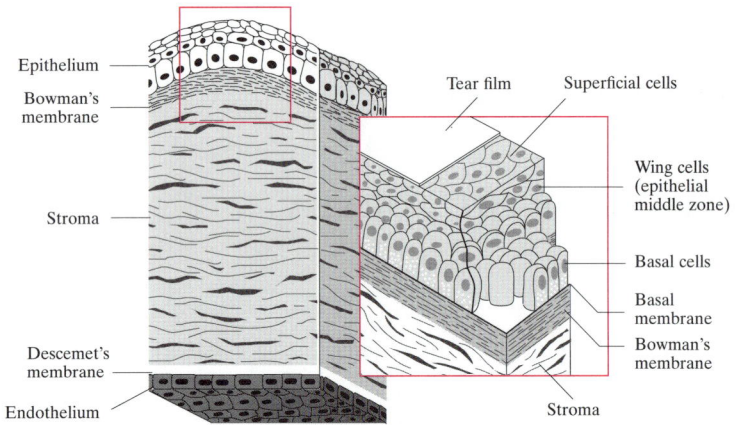

HEREDITARY CORNEAL DYSTROPHIES

ANTERIOR CORNEAL DYSTROPHIES

Features	Map–dot–fingerprint dystrophy (Cogan's microcystic, epithelial basement membrane)	Reis-Bücklers' dystrophy	Hereditary juvenile epithelial dystrophy (Meesmann's)	Anterior mosaic degeneration (crocodile shagreen)
Inheritance	Autosomal dominant	Autosomal dominant	Autosomal dominant	Autosomal dominant
Presentation	Middle age; recurrent epithelial erosions	Early childhood; recurrent epithelial erosions, reduced vision	Very early childhood; mild irritation	Incidental finding; usually asymptomatic
Biomicroscopy	Geographic map, dot, fingerprint or cystic appearance	Cloudy Bowman's membrane; ring-shaped honeycomb appearance; corneal periphery is spared	Intraepithelial microcysts with clear surrounding epithelium	Grey cloudiness in the central cornea at the level of Bowman's membrane or more posteriorly (posterior crocodile shagreen)

STROMAL DYSTROPHIES

Features	Granular dystrophy	Lattice dystrophy	Macular dystrophy	Central crystalline dystrophy (Schnyder's)
Inheritance	Autosomal dominant	Autosomal dominant	Autosomal recessive	Autosomal dominant
Age of onset	First decade of life	End of first decade of life	First two decades of life	First decade of life
Symptoms	Usually asymptomatic; visual acuity deteriorates with age	Recurrent corneal erosions; visual deterioration; association with systemic amyloidosis in type II	Mild recurrent corneal erosions; early visual deterioration	Usually no significant visual loss; may be associated with hyper-lipidaemia
Corneal opacity	Clear areas between the lesions; no peripheral involvement	Corneal periphery remains clear	Extension to the periphery and from anterior to posterior stroma over time	Central corneal involvement at the level of the anterior stroma
Pathology	Hyaline deposits	Amyloid deposition	Glycosaminoglycan deposits	Cholesterol crystals

BIOMICROSCOPIC PRESENTATION OF CORNEAL AND ENDOTHELIAL DYSTROPHIES

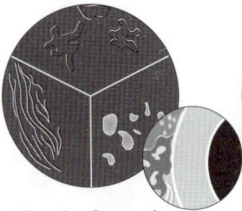

Map–dot-fingerprint dystrophy

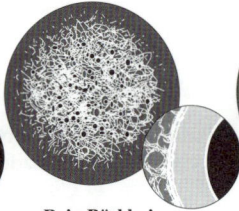

Reis–Bückler's dystrophy

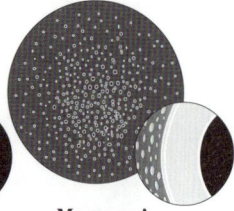

Meesmann's dystrophy

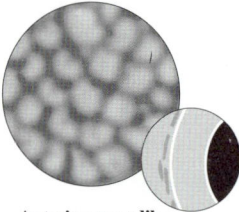

Anterior crocodile shagreen degeneration

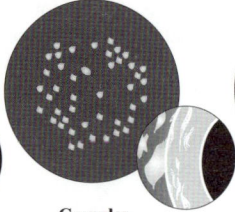

Granular dystrophy

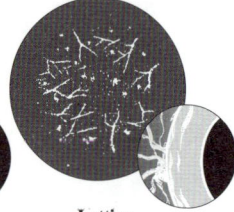

Lattice dystrophy

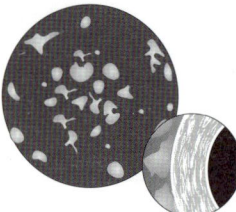

Macular dystrophy

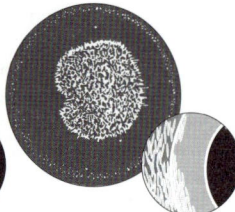

Schnyder's crystalline dystrophy

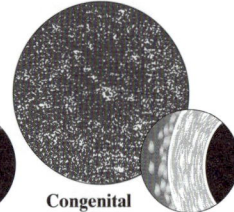

Congenital hereditary endothelial dystrophy

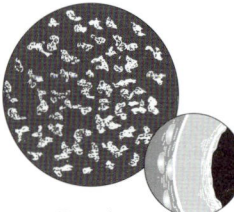

Posterior polymorphous dystrophy

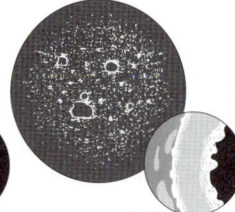

Fuchs' endothelial dystrophy

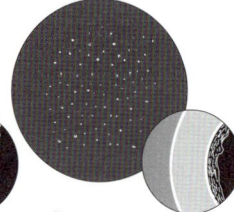

Cornea guttata

ENDOTHELIAL DYSTROPHIES

CLINICAL FEATURES OF ENDOTHELIAL DYSTROPHIES

Features	Congenital hereditary endothelial dystrophy		Posterior polymorphous dystrophy	Fuchs' endothelial dystrophy
Inheritance	Autosomal recessive	Autosomal dominant	Autosomal dominant, recessive, sporadic	Autosomal dominant, sporadic
Laterality	Bilateral	Bilateral	Bilateral or unilateral	Bilateral
Age of onset	At birth	1–2 years of life	At birth or in the first year of life	Middle age or later
Signs and symptoms	None	Photophobia, tearing	Angle changes, glaucoma	Oedema, pain
Progression	Minimal	Slow progressive	Slow progressive	Slow progressive
Corneal thickness	Thickened (2–3-fold)	Thickened (2–3-fold)	Normal or thickened	Mild (2-fold) thickened
Corneal opacifications	Diffuse, ground-glass appearance	Diffuse, ground-glass appearance	Isolated or diffuse lesions with a vesicular, curvilinear appearance	Central, paracentral oedema
Nystagmus	Common	Rare	Very rare	None

ENDOTHELIAL DEGENERATION

CAUSES OF ENDOTHELIAL DEGENERATION

Pseudophakic bullous keratopathy
Aphakic bullous keratopathy
Bullous keratopathy due to raised IOP
• untreated angle closure glaucoma
• buphthalmos
Bullous keratopathy following trauma
Toxic bullous keratopathy
Inflammatory bullous keratopathy in uveitis
Keratopathy in prolonged contact lens wear

RECURRENT CORNEAL EROSIONS

Primary epithelial disease

Map–dot–fingerprint dystrophy
Meesmann's dystrophy

Secondary epithelial disease

Facial palsy (neuroparalytic keratitis)
Trigeminal nerve lesion (neurotrophic keratitis)
Following infection (herpes simplex, zoster, bacteria, fungi, acanthamoeba)
Keratoconjunctivitis sicca, Sjögren's syndrome, eyelid anomalies
Graft versus host disease
Prolonged contact lens wear keratopathy
Rosacea blepharoconjunctivitis

Primary basement membrane disease

Diabetes mellitus
Reis–Bückler's dystrophy

Secondary basement membrane disease

Trauma

Combined epithelial and basement membrane disorders

Chemical injury, radiation burns
Collagen diseases
Pemphigoid, erythema multiforme
Keratomalacia

CORNEAL DEPOSITION

Aetiology (disease, intra-ocular foreign body, drug)	Corneal deposition
Wilson's disease (hepatolenticular degeneration)	Green ring (Kayser–Fleischer ring) in the peripheral deep stroma and Descemet's membrane
Hypercalcaemia	Calcium deposits
Mucopolysaccharidoses	Corneal depositions may occur in all mucopolysaccharidoses (except Sanfilippo's syndrome)

Aetiology (disease, intra-ocular foreign body, drug)	Corneal deposition
Hurler's, Scheie's, Morquio's, Maroteaux–Lamy's and Sly's syndromes	Variable degrees of corneal clouding which usually occur early in life (corneal clouding may require penetrating keratoplasty; in Hurler's syndrome, the corneal changes may include oedema secondary to glaucoma)
Hunter's syndrome	Corneal clouding occurs late in life or remains absent
Cystinosis	Glittering crystals in the anterior cornea
Alkaptonuria	Dark pigmentation
Gout	Urate crystals
Fabry's disease and drug-related (e.g. amiodarone)	Cornea verticillata (vortex keratopathy)
Silver	Argyrosis (stroma and Descemet's membrane)
Copper	Green–blue deposits, chalcosis
Iron	Brown deposition, siderosis (stroma)
Iron	Hudson–Stähli line in the epithelium (age-related)
Pterygium	Stocker's line (epithelial iron deposition adjacent to pterygium)
Filter blister	Ferry's line (epithelial iron deposition anterior to filter blister)
Gold	Chrysiasis (posterior stroma)
Phenothiazines	Pigmented lines (deep stroma)

BAND KERATOPATHY

CAUSES OF BAND KERATOPATHY

Hypercalcaemia	Sarcoidosis
	Uraemia, hyperparathyroidism
	Hyperphosphataemia
	Plasmocytoma
	Discoid lupus erythematosus
	Vitamin D intoxication
	Lung and bone metastases
	Ichthyosis
Gout	Hyperuricaemia
Ocular disease	Chronic uveitis (in juvenile rheumatoid arthritis)
	Long-standing raised IOP, longstanding corneal oedema
	Phthisis bulbi
	Spheroidal degeneration
	Norrie's disease (Andersen–Warburg syndrome)

Chronic exposure
  to mercurial
  vapours
Labrador
  keratopathy
  (climate-
  related)
Dry eye
Idiopathic

PERIPHERAL CORNEAL ULCERATION

PERIPHERAL CORNEAL ULCERATIONS AND UNDERLYING PATHOLOGY

Ocular, infectious	Microbial keratitis (hypersensitivity reaction)
Ocular, non-infectious	Mooren's ulcer
	Terrien's marginal degeneration
Systemic, infectious	Bacterial dysentery, AIDS, tuberculosis, gonorrhoea, syphilis
Systemic, non-infectious	Collagen disease: rheumatoid arthritis, disseminated lupus erythematosus, scleroderma, polyarteritis nodosa, temporal arteritis, Wegener's granulomatosis, recurrent polychondritis
	Acute leukaemia
	Behçet's disease, sarcoidosis, rosacea
	Gold intoxication

BACTERIAL KERATITIS

TYPICAL CORNEAL RESPONSES TO CERTAIN ORGANISMS

Staphylococcus aureus, ***Pneumococcus***	Oval, yellow–white, densely opaque suppuration surrounded by clear cornea
Pseudomonas	Irregular, sharply demarcated ulceration with surrounding stromal oedema, mucopurulent discharge, impending perforation
Enterobacteria (*Escherichia coli*, *Proteus*, Klebsiella, *Serratia marcescens*)	Grey–white suppuration with diffuse stromal opacity, ring-shaped infiltrates (hypersensitivity reaction)

KERATOMYCOSIS

CLINICAL FEATURES OF KERATOMYCOSIS (FUNGAL KERATITIS)

- Map-like corneal infiltrates
- Superficial epithelial defect

- Isolated or multifocal poorly defined infiltrates
- Infiltrates may have filamentous edges
- A hypopyon may be present

TREATMENT OF CANDIDA KERATITIS

Topical (hourly)	Miconazole 10% Amphotericin B 0.15%
Subconjunctival injection	Miconazole 5–10 mg
Systemic	Flunconazole 200 mg twice daily Ketoconazole 200 mg twice daily

HERPES KERATITIS

ANTERIOR SEGMENT MANIFESTATIONS OF HERPETIC EYE DISEASE

I.	**Primary infection**	Neonatal Primary (children and adults)
II.	**Recurrent infection**	Blepharitis Conjunctivitis Keratitis Keratouveitis Trabeculitis Iridocyclitis

RECURRENT HERPES SIMPLEX KERATITIS

I. Epithelial keratitis
Punctate keratitis
Dendritic keratitis
Geographic ulcer

II. Metaherpetic keratitis, trophic corneal ulcer

III. Stromal (immunological) keratitis
  1. Antigen–antibody–complement-mediated
   Interstitial keratitis
   Wessely's immune rings
   Limbal vasculitis
  2. Lymphocyte-mediated
   Nonnecrotizing disciform keratitis
   Endothelitis

SIDE-EFFECTS OF TOPICAL ANTIVIRAL AGENTS

Eyelids	Swelling or occlusion of the lacrimal gland Swelling or occlusion of Meibomian glands Ptosis (Delayed) allergic reaction

Conjunctiva   Hyperaemia, chemosis
Follicular conjunctivitis
Limbal oedema

Cornea   Superficial punctate keratitis
Superficial pannus formation
Filamentary keratopathy
Delayed wound healing of epithelial and stromal ulcerations

TREATMENT OF HERPETIC KERATITIS

Epithelial keratitis

	Debridement by wiping	Topical anaesthetic is instilled into the lower fornix; affected epithelium is then removed with a cotton wool applicator and sent to the virology department for confirmation of diagnosis
	Antiviral drugs	Acyclovir eye ointment (3%) 5 times daily, continued until the third day after corneal healing
		Trifluorothymidine 1% eye drops every two hours in the first two days, then four times daily for two weeks*
		Adenine arabinoside eye drops or ointment for resistant cases*
• in **co-existing iritis**	Mydriatic	Atropine 1%, once or twice daily
• in **extensive ulcerations** with possible super-infection	Antibiotics	Tetracycline eye ointment, for example

Disciform keratitis

	Steroid eye drops	Dexamethasone eye drops 2–4 times daily
	Mydriatic	Atropine 1%, once or twice daily

Antiviral drugs	Acyclovir eye ointment (3%) 5 times daily

Necrotizing stromal keratitis

Antiviral therapy	Acyclovir eye ointment (3%) and oral acyclovir 400 (–800) mg 5 times daily
Topical steroids	Four times daily, 2–3 days after commencement of antiviral therapy
Bandage contact lens	May be used instead of padding

Recurrent corneal erosions, trophic ulcer
(if healing not achieved with conventional treatment within one week)

Bandage contact lens (with high water content)	
Antibiotics	e.g. gentamicin eye drops twice daily
Lubricants (without preservatives)	Four times daily, more frequent if needed

Zoster ophthalmicus (with corneal involvement)

Antiviral therapy	Acyclovir eye ointment (3%) and oral acyclovir 800 mg 5 times daily for 5–7 days
Steroids	Prednisolone 30–60 mg daily may prevent zoster neuralgia

* Not universally available

CHEMICAL/THERMAL BURNS

IMMEDIATE TREATMENT OF CHEMICAL/THERMAL BURNS

Copious self-irrigation of the affected eye using the nearest source of water should be started as soon as possible. After arrival at the accident and emergency department, topical anaesthetic should be applied to reduce the patient's discomfort and to overcome orbicularis spasm. The eyelids should be held apart and irrigation is continued with normal saline 0.9% or a chemical neutralizing solution until the conjuctival pH normalizes. Double evertion of the upper lid should be performed to enable proper evaluation of the superior fornix. Cotton wool applicators should be used to remove chemical particles. In alkali burns, ethylenediamine tetraacetate (EDTA; edetic acid) solution may be used as an additional irrigant.

FURTHER TREATMENT OF CHEMICAL/THERMAL BURNS

- Topical antibiotics to prevent infection
- Topical mydriatic (e.g. cyclopentolate)
- Vitamin C 1000–2000 mg daily
- Oral carbonic anhydrase inhibitors in uncontrolled IOP
- Indomethacin or diclofenac 50–100 mg twice daily
- Systemic analgesia if needed
- Eye pad (not in alkali burns)
- Daily ophthalmic review (especially in alkali burns)
- Sodium hyaluronate can be applied on cornea and conjunctiva for surface protection in severe cases
- Bandage contact lens or tarsorrhaphy may be needed
- Epithelial transplantation if incomplete corneal regeneration after 2–3 weeks

Alkali burns may need

- topical steroids
- topical vitamin C as well as antibiotics, mydriatics and oral vitamin C, and preservative-free drops may be considered if they are to be used frequently

GRADING OF CHEMICAL/THERMAL BURNS

I   Erosion, hyperaemia, no ischaemia (good prognosis)
II   Ischaemia in $<\frac{1}{3}$ of the limbus, iris details not obscured (good prognosis)
III Ischaemia in between $\frac{1}{3}$ and $\frac{1}{2}$ of the limbus, complete epithelial loss, poor view of iris details (guarded prognosis)
IV   Ischaemia in $>\frac{1}{2}$ of the limbus, dense corneal opacification, extensive necrosis, extensive ulceration, iris atrophy, cataract, glaucoma (poor prognosis)

KERATOPLASTY

INDICATIONS FOR KERATOPLASTY

Optical   Corneal opacities
                 Keratoconus
Therapeutic Deep keratitis: granulomatous reaction at the level of
                 Descemet's membrane in herpetic keratitis
                 Primary or secondary endothelial decompensation
                 Perforated corneal ulcers
Tectonic   Post-operative fistula following intra-ocular surgery
                 Following tumour removal

External fistula in necrotic wounds
Anterior segment reconstruction
Posttraumatic corneal defects

RISK FACTORS FOR GRAFT REJECTION

1. Vascularization of the host cornea
2. Loosening of suture induces vascularization
3. Absent Bowman's lamella predisposes to loosening of suture
4. Anterior synechiae at the graft margin
5. Endothelial decompensation predisposes to vascularization
6. Large graft diameter (>7.5 mm)
7. Repeated grafting (sensitization)

REMOVAL OF SUTURES

• Not earlier than one year postoperatively
• In Fuchs' dystrophy or in herpes simplex stromal keratitis after 1.5–2
  years

CORNEAL REFRACTIVE SURGERY

The corneal refractive power is appproximately two-thirds of the total
refractive power of the eye. This provides the basis for corneal refractive
surgery: a relatively small change in the corneal curvature causes a significant
change in the refractive status of the eye.

The three surgical categories of corrective corneal refractive surgery are
incisional surgery, lamellar surgery and thermokeratoplasty.

INCISIONAL SURGERY

Radial keratotomy

Four or eight partial-thickness radial incisions are made in the peripheral
cornea. They weaken the cornea and cause central flattening. The central
cornea remains clear. Radial keratotomy is a relatively quick and inexpensive
surgical procedure to correct myopia. It can be combined with transverse
posterior keratotomy to correct coexisting astigmatism. However, intersecting
incisions should be avoided.

Astigmatic keratotomy

Transverse keratotomy

Transverse or arcuate incisions are placed along the steepest meridian to
flatten it. Various techniques and nomograms exist.

Wedge resection

In high astigmatism, a corneal wedge can be excised from the flattest
meridian. Tightening sutures will cause steepening of this meridian.

Hexagonal keratotomy

Six transverse, paracentral corneal incisions induce a forward shift of the central cornea for hypermetropia correction. Multiple postoperative complications have been reported, and some surgeons have advised that the procedure should not be used.

LAMELLAR PROCEDURES

Keratomileusis

A microkeratome is used to perform a central lamellar keratectomy. The posterior aspect of the resected disc is resurfaced for correction of myopia (central flattening) or hypermetropia (peripheral flattening with compensatory central steepening). Automated lamellar keratectomy (ALK) and excimer laser-assisted *in situ* keratomileusis (LASIK) are recent developments.

Keratophakia

An intrastromal inlay (donor cornea or synthetic material) is used to increase the refractive power of the cornea for correction of hypermetropia.

Epikeratoplasty

Prelathed donor cornea is used as a 'permanent contact lens' sutured onto the recipient de-epithelialized cornea. Disappointing results and numerous post-operative complications have been reported.

Excimer laser photo-refractive keratectomy (PRK)

Excimer laser high-precision surface ablation, or more recently indirect intrastromal ablation, are becoming increasingly popular methods for correction of refractive errors. However, they remain expensive procedures and long-term results are still under investigation.

THERMOKERATOPLASTY

Heat or more recently holmium laser are used to cause peripheral collagen shrinkage to induce central steepening for correction of hypermetropia.

EPISCLERITIS, SCLERITIS

CLASSIFICATION OF NONINFECTIOUS SCLERITIS AND EPISCLERITIS

[Watson PG (1980) The diagnoses and management of scleritis. *Ophthalmology* **87**:716–720]

Episcleritis

Simple episcleritis
Nodular episcleritis

Scleritis

Anterior scleritis

- Non-necrotizing
  Nodular
  Diffuse
- Necrotizing (with/without inflammation)

Posterior scleritis

EPISCLERITIS VERSUS SCLERITIS

	Episcleritis	Scleritis
Onset	Sudden (within 24 hours)	Gradual (over days)
Laterality	Unilateral	Unilateral or bilateral
Pain	Foreign body sensation, mild tenderness to touch	Gnawing pain which may radiate peri-bulbarly

SYMPTOMS OF POSTERIOR SCLERITIS

- Deep orbital pain with peribulbar radiation
- Visual impairment
- Radiographic signs (scleral thickening distinguishable on CT; demonstration of Tenon space with B-scan ultrasonography)
- Variable symptoms
  Fundal changes
      Exudative detachment
      Sectorial or circular choroidal detachment
      Papilloedema
      Macular oedema
  Visual field changes
  Anterior chamber flattening
  Exophthalmos
  Restricted ocular motility
  Palpebral swelling or retraction
  Enlargement of the sub-Tenon space

Chapter 6

GLAUCOMA/IRIS

AQUEOUS HUMOUR/RECEPTORS IN THE ANTERIOR PART OF THE EYE

COMPOSITION OF NORMAL AQUEOUS HUMOUR IN RELATION TO PLASMA

Slightly hyperosmotic, acid pH
High ascorbate content
Excess of Cl^- and lactic acid
Slight excess of Na^+
Deficit of bicarbonate, carbon dioxide and glucose
Other substances: amino acids (variable concentrations), hyaluronic acid,
traces of the components of the coagulation and fibrinolytic systems
(plasminogen and plasminogen proactivator are present in more significant
amounts), small amounts of lens crystallines (the concentration increases in
the presence of a cataract)

THE RECEPTORS IN THE ANTERIOR PART OF THE EYE

Receptor	Location	Action	Drug
Adrenergic neurones			
α_1 receptors	Dilator pupillae muscle	Mydriasis, increase in the facility of aqueous outflow	Guanethidine (acts indirectly)
β_2 receptors	Trabecular meshwork	Increase in the facility of aqueous outflow	Adrenaline derivatives
β_2 receptors	Ciliary epithelia	Receptor block decreases aqueous secretion	Beta-blockers
Cholinergic neurones			
Muscarine receptors	Ciliary muscle and sphincter pupillae muscle	Contraction of the ciliary muscle, increase in the facility of the aqueous outflow	Parasympathomimetics

EXAMINATION OF THE ANGLE

ANATOMY OF THE ANGLE

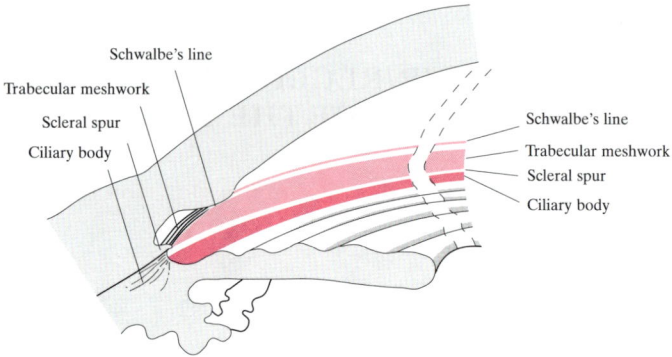

SCHEIE'S SYSTEM FOR RECORDING OF GONIOSCOPIC ANGLE GRADING

[Scheie HG (1957) Width and pigmentation of the angle of the anterior chamber. A system of grading by gonioscopy. *Arch Ophthalmol* **58**:510–512]

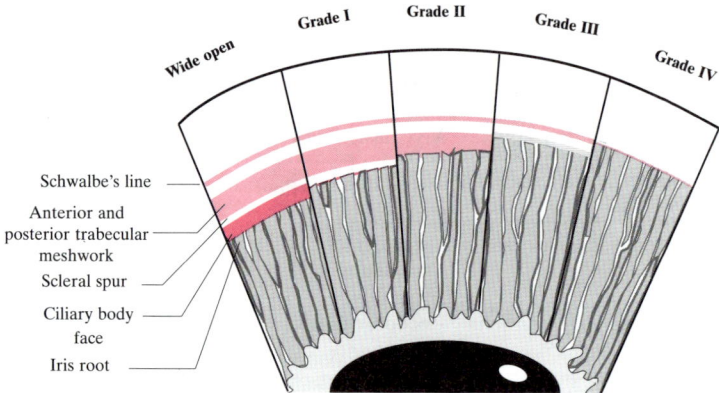

Wide open		All the structures of the angle visible
Slightly narrowed	Grade I	Minimal view of the ciliary body face
Narrow	Grade II	Ciliary body face not visible
Narrow	Grade III	Posterior half of the trabeculum not visible
Narrow/closed	Grade IV	Only Schwalbe's line or none of the angle is visible

SHAFFER'S SYSTEM FOR RECORDING OF GONIOSCOPIC ANGLE GRADING

[Shaffer RN (1960) Symposium: primary glaucomas III. Gonioscopy, ophthalmoscopy and perimetry. *Trans Am Acad Ophthalmol Otolaryngol* **62**:112–127]

Angle width	Risk of closure
Wide open (20–45°)	Nil

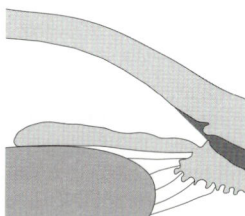

Narrow (10–20°)	Possible

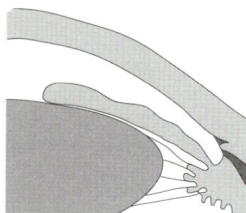

Very narrow (less than 10°)	Likely

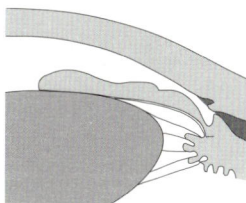

Iridocorneal contact (0°)	Closed angle

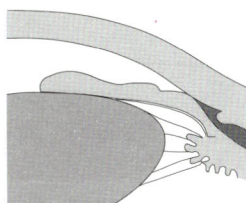

ESTIMATION OF THE DEPTH OF THE PERIPHERAL ANTERIOR CHAMBER

VAN HERICK'S SYSTEM OF ANGLE ESTIMATION

[Van Herick W, Shaffer RN, Schwartz A (1969) Estimation of width of angle of anterior chamber. *Am J Ophthalmol* **68**:626]

The Van Herick method uses the slit lamp to estimate the width of the angle:
1. A narrow slit beam is placed perpendicular to the most peripheral part of the cornea.
2. The eye pieces are placed at an angle of 60° from the light beam.
3. The corneal thickness (CT) is used to estimate the anterior chamber depth (ACD).

Grade 1   ACD less than $\frac{1}{4}$ CT

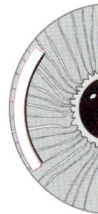

Grade 2   ACD = $\frac{1}{4}$ CT

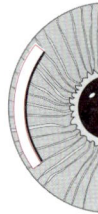

Grade 3   ACD = $\frac{1}{4}$ to $\frac{1}{2}$ CT

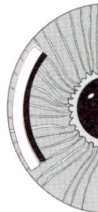

Grade 4   ACD same or more than CT

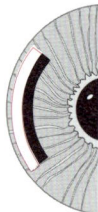

SCHIÖTZ TONOMETER

CALIBRATION TABLE FOR SCHIÖTZ TONOMETER (1955)

Reading	5.5 g	7.5 g	10.0 g
0	41	59	82
0.5	38	54	75
1.0	34.5	50	69
1.5	32	46	64
2.0	29	42	59
2.5	26.5	39	55
3.0	24	36	51
3.5	22	33	47
4.0	20.5	30	43
4.5	19	28	40
5.0	17	26	37
5.5	16	24	34
6.0	14.5	22	32
6.5	13	20	29
7.0	12	18.5	27
7.5	11	17	25
8.0	10	16	23
8.5	9	14	21
9.0	8.5	13	19.5
9.5	8	12	18
10.0	7	11	16.5
11.0	6	9	14
12.0	4.9	7.5	11.5
13.0	4	6.2	9.5
14.0		5	7.8
15.0		4	6.4

Documentation of measurement with the Schiötz tonometer
For example:

Scale reading: 5
Weight carried by plunger: 5.5 g
(Friedenwald 1955 nomogram indicates IOP of 17 mmHg)

is recorded as

$$5/5.5 = 17 \, \text{mmHg} \, (\text{'}55)$$

TONOGRAPHY

ESTIMATION OF TOTAL AQUEOUS OUTFLOW FACILITY

Grant formula: $C = \dfrac{\Delta V}{t(\Delta p)}$

C Coefficient of the facility of aqueous outflow (μl/min per mmHg)
ΔV Change in the aqueous volume (μl)
t Time (min)
Δp Change in intraocular pressure during four continuous minutes (mmHg)

The intraocular pressure is read in mmHg from an electronic Schiötz scale, which replaces the scale of the hand-held Schiötz tonometer. By convention, the usual tonographic time period is 4 min ($t = 4$) and the readings are recorded as a graph showing the change in intraocular tension (Δp). The aqueous volume loss from the eye is determined by the Friedenwald nomogram (ΔV). The facility of aqueous outflow (C) is determined by the Grant formula. The median coefficient of the facility of aqueous outflow is 0.28 μl/min per mmHg.

Elevated coefficient of outflow in normal intraocular pressure

- Increased friction by the plunger
- Low ocular rigidity
- Hyposecretion of aqueous humour

Elevated coefficient of outflow in elevated intraocular pressure

- initial intraocular pressure artificially elevated (e.g. due to digital compression of the globe)
- high ocular rigidity
- high pseudofacility (due to decreased aqueous secretion)
- increased episcleral venous pressure
- closed angle glaucoma (the tonometer weight can lead to opening of the angle)
- Moses effect (due to indentation of the cornea in the space between the plunger and the opening of the tonometer footplate in electronic tonometers)

GLAUCOMATOUS DISC CHANGES

DISC CHANGES INDICATIVE OF SUSPECTED GLAUCOMA

- documented progressive enlargement of the cup
- narrow neuroretinal rims
- nerve fibre bundle defects
- asymmetrical cup (difference of more than 0.2 in the c/d ratio★)
- large excavation (c/d ratio★ >0.6)
- splinter-shaped haemorrhage on the disc margin
- asymmetry in the cup shape
- pallor of the optic nerve head cup
- visibility of the lamina cribrosa

- asymmetrical expansion in the vertical sectors of the cup
- nasal displacement of the central blood vessels
- bayonetting of the vessels
- peripapillary atrophy

PERIPAPILLARY CHOROIDAL ATROPHY ZONES

Zone	Ophthalmoscopy	Histology	Perimetry
α	Irregular hypo- and hyperpigmentation	Pigment and structure irregularity of the retinal pigment epithelium	Relative scotoma
β	Visible large choroidal vessels or visible sclera	Loss of retinal pigment epithelium cells with exposed Bruch membrane	Absolute scotoma

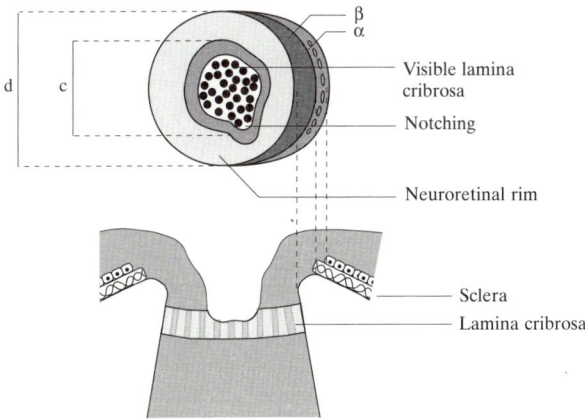

* The estimation of the so-called cup/disc ratio is the diameter of the cup (*c*) expressed as a fraction of the diameter of the disc (*d*) in the vertical meridian (*c/d* ratio in the above illustration is approximately 0.6)

VISUAL FIELD DEFECTS IN GLAUCOMA

THE FOUR TYPES OF COMPLETE NERVE FIBRE BUNDLES DEFECTS

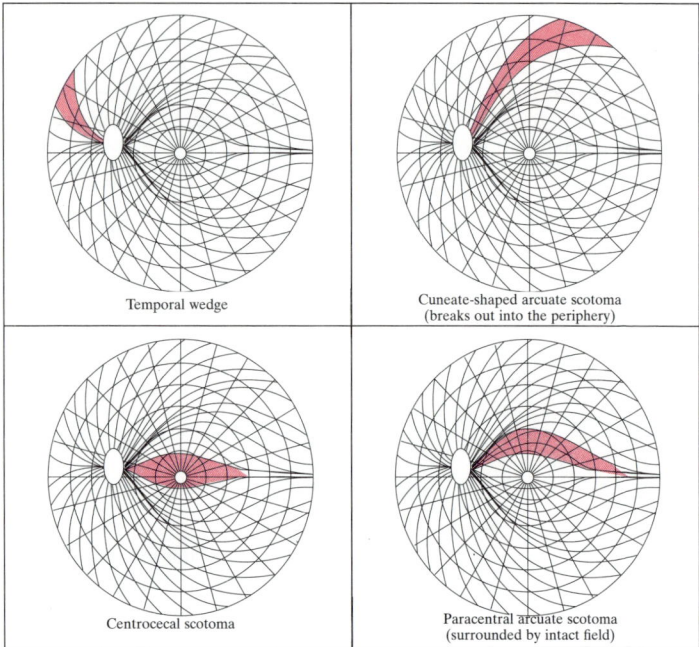

Temporal wedge

Cuneate-shaped arcuate scotoma
(breaks out into the periphery)

Centrocecal scotoma

Paracentral arcuate scotoma
(surrounded by intact field)

TYPICAL EARLY GLAUCOMATOUS VISUAL FIELD DEFECTS
IN MANUAL PERIMETRY

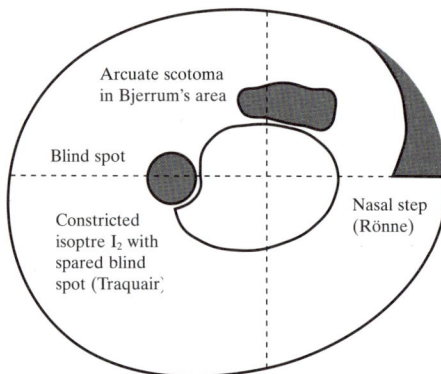

Arcuate scotoma
in Bjerrum's area

Blind spot

Constricted
isoptre I_2 with
spared blind
spot (Traquair)

Nasal step
(Rönne)

PROGRESSION OF GLAUCOMATOUS VISUAL FIELD DEFECTS

[Aulhorn E, Karmeyer H (1977) Frequency distribution in early glaucomatous visual field defects. *Doc Ophthalmol Proc Ser* **14**:75–83]

Stages of glaucomatous usual field defects

I. Relative scotoma

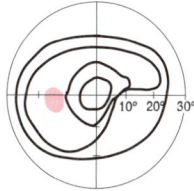

II. Absolute defects not connected to the blind spot

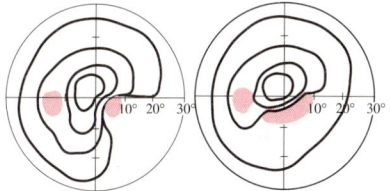

III. Absolute arcuate scotoma extending to the blind spot (with possible nasal break-out)

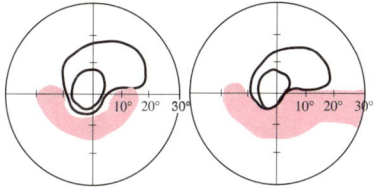

IV. Extended absolute arcuate scotoma (altitudinal defect)

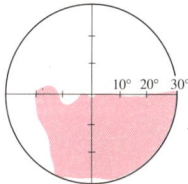

V. Extended absolute scotoma with residual temporal field

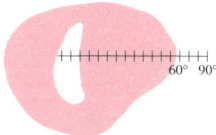

GLAUCOMA: CLASSIFICATION

CLASSIFICATION OF THE VARIOUS GLAUCOMAS ACCORDING TO
UNDERLYING PHYSIOLOGICAL MECHANISM

I. Open-angle glaucoma

A. *Primary open-angle glaucoma*

B. *Secondary open-angle glaucoma*

1. Pretrabecular
2. Trabecular
   a. Accumulation of extracellular material
   b. Structural changes
3. Posttrabecular

C. *Congenital open-angle glaucoma*

1. Primary congenital glaucoma
2. Congenital glaucoma with other anomalies

II. Angle-closure glaucoma

A. *Primary angle-closure glaucoma*

B. *Secondary angle-closure glaucoma*

1. Anterior type (iris pulled over the trabecular meshwork)
2. Posterior type (iris pushed over the trabecular meshwork)
   a. with pupillary block
   b. without pupillary block
   c. congenital angle-closure glaucoma

```
                          ┌──────────────┐
                          │ Intraocular  │
                          │  pressure    │
                          └──────────────┘
              ┌──────────────────┴────────────────────┐
        ┌──────────┐                              ┌──────────┐
        │ Elevated │                              │  Within  │
        └──────────┘                              │  normal  │
    ┌────────┴────────┐                           │  limits  │
                                                  └──────────┘
┌─────────────┐ ┌──────────────────────┐ ┌──────────────────┐
│Normal visual│ │ Normal visual fields │ │  Glaucomatous    │
│fields,      │ │ or visual field      │ │  visual field    │
│normal optic │ │ defects, glaucomatous│ │  defects,        │
│nerve head   │ │ optic nerve disc,    │ │  glaucomatous    │
│             │ │ nerve fibre bundle   │ │  optic nerve     │
│             │ │ defects              │ │  disc            │
└─────────────┘ └──────────────────────┘ └──────────────────┘
┌─────────────┐ ┌──────────────────────┐ ┌──────────────────┐
│Ocular       │ │   Glaucoma           │ │  Low-tension     │
│hyperten-    │ │   (likely)           │ │  glaucoma        │
│sion, or     │ │                      │ │                  │
│early        │ │                      │ │                  │
│glaucoma     │ │                      │ │                  │
└─────────────┘ └──────────────────────┘ └──────────────────┘
              ┌──────────────────┐
              │ Possible secondary│
              │ glaucoma to be    │
              │ excluded          │
              └──────────────────┘
```

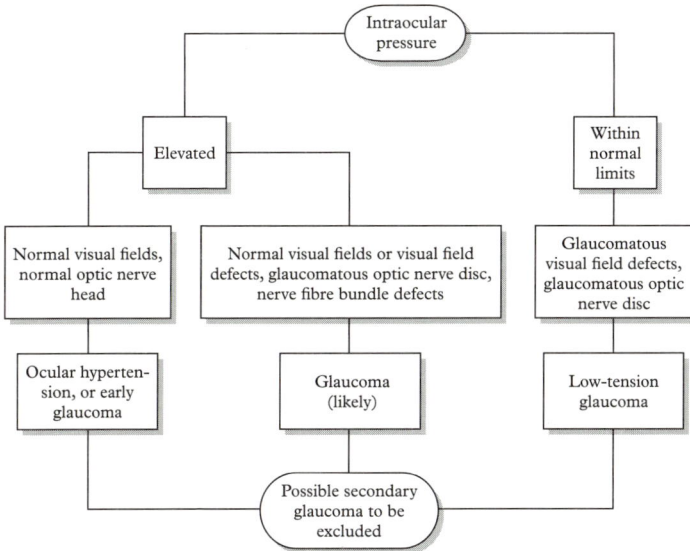

SECONDARY GLAUCOMA

Condition	Characteristic features
Glaucoma in developmental anomalies	
Iridocorneal dysgenesis (Axenfeld's, Reiger's and Peter's anomalies)	Congenital iridocorneal malformations
Aniridia	Angle anomaly (associated glaucoma in 50% of cases
Trabecular-block open-angle glaucoma	
Pseudo-exfoliation glaucoma	Grey dandruff-like material throughout the anterior segment of the eye, but none present in the mid-lenticular zone due to constant rubbing of the pupil; characteristic gonioscopic findings include an hyperpigmented angle and Sampaolesi's line anterior to Schwalbe's line
Pigment dispersion syndrome glaucoma	Krukenberg's spindle on the corneal endothelium; transillumination of the iris; heavily pigmented angle
Steroid-induced glaucoma	5% of the general population are high responders (markedly elevated IOP after 4–6 weeks)

Glaucoma in corneal endothelial abnormalities

Iridocorneal endothelial (ICE) syndromes (Chandler's and Cogan–Reese syndromes, essential iris atrophy)	Secondary angle-closure glaucoma due to peripheral anterior synechiae
Posterior polymorphous dystrophy	Rare hereditary dystrophy with thickening of the posterior lamellae of Descemet's membrane and atypical cells on the corneal endothelium; glaucoma in approximately 15% of cases

Lens-related glaucoma

Phacomorphic glaucoma	Pupillary block in intumescent lens
Glaucoma in dislocated crystalline lens (ectopia lentis, Marfan's syndrome, Weill–Marchesani syndrome, homocystinuria)	Glaucoma due to pupillary block
Phacolytic glaucoma	Secondary open-angle glaucoma due to trabecular block with lens proteins and macrophages
Retained lens matter glaucoma	May occur after cataract surgery or lens injury

Retinal ischaemia glaucoma

Neovascular glaucoma	Secondary angle closure due to fibrovascular membranes; commonest causes are central retinal vein occlusion and diabetes mellitus

Posttraumatic glaucoma

Red cell glaucoma	Secondary angle closure due to trabeculum obstructing red blood cells following traumatic hyphaema
Chronic erythroclastic glaucoma	Secondary angle closure due to trabeculum obstructing degenerated red blood cells (ghost cells) in prolonged hyphaema or more commonly after vitreous haemorrhages
Angle-recession glaucoma	Late-onset glaucoma due to trabecular injury after blunt ocular trauma

SECONDARY GLAUCOMA

Condition	Characteristic features
Glaucoma due to intraocular inflammation	
Acute uveitis	Outflow obstruction, on the one hand, and later topical steroid-induced increased aqueous production, on the other hand, leading to elevation of intra-ocular pressure
Chronic uveitis	Glaucoma due to indirect changes in the angle (anterior synechiae)
Fuchs' heterochromic cyclitis	Small keratic precipitates scattered throughout the corneal endothelium; absence of posterior synechiae; the affected eye is hypochromic, although in some cases heterochromia may be absent; topical steroids usually do not improve the cyclitis; manifestation of open-angle glaucoma is thought to be due to trabecular sclerosis and may also be related to the use of topical steroids in some patients; trabeculectomy with 5-fluorouracil is often needed to control the intraocular pressure
Glaucomatocyclitic crisis (Posner–Schlossman syndrome)	Unilateral, recurrent anterior uveitis with markedly raised intraocular pressure but usually painless
Elevated episcleral venous pressure	
Carotid-cavernous fistula	The venous pressure in an arteriovenous fistula between the carotid artery and the cavernous sinus is raised. The rise in episcleral venous pressure may lead to elevated intraocular pressure
Sturge–Weber syndrome	Secondary glaucoma due to episcleral haemangioma and raised episcleral venous pressure occurs in about one-third of cases; facial angioma and ipsilateral angioma of the meninges and brain are common; an eye with upper lid angioma is at increased risk of glaucoma
Orbital space-occupying lesions (tumours, endocrine orbitopathy, orbital varices)	Abnormal venous outflow
Glaucoma in ocular tumours	
Uveal melanoma	Direct trabecular block due to presence of the lesion in the angle or indirect involvement due to trabecular block with tumour cells, pigment granules or macrophages

Ocular tumours in children (retinoblastoma, juvenile xanthogranuloma, medulloepithelioma)	Possible secondary glaucoma due to iridal changes or neovascularization

Glaucoma following intraocular surgery

Encircling buckle	May cause elevated intraocular pressure due to raised episcleral venous pressure
Silicone oil intravitreal injection	Rise of intraocular pressure may occur due to silicone oil in the anterior chamber causing trabecular block or due to the high viscosity silicone oil pushing the lens against the iris causing pupillary block
Aphakia or pseudophakia	Various pathogenetic mechanisms, e.g. vitreous herniation into the anterior chamber causing trabecular block, residual viscoelastic substance transiently blocking the aqueous outflow system, chronic peripheral anterior synechiae or intra-ocular lens-induced pupillary block
Malignant glaucoma	Flattening of the anterior chamber and closure of the angle due to vitreous expansion; most common after glaucoma surgery but also after cataract removal procedures

NEOVASCULAR GLAUCOMA

CAUSES OF NEOVASCULAR GLAUCOMA

- Diabetic retinopathy (~30% of cases)
- Retinal vein occlusion (~30% of cases)
- Other retinal causes
    Retinal artery occlusion
    Long-standing retinal detachment
    Intraocular tumours (retinoblastona, Von Hippel–Lindau's syndrome, malignant melanoma, choroidal metastasis)
    Sickle cell anaemia
    Coats' disease
    Eales' disease
    Retinopathy of prematurity
    Retinoschisis
    Stickler's syndrome
    Norrie's disease
- Other ocular causes
    Uveitis
    Endophthalmitis
    Silicone oil-induced

Post-operative ischaemia of the anterior segment
Long-standing uncontrolled Intra-ocular pressure in primary open-angle glaucoma
Chronic ocular ischaemia
- Extraocular vascular causes
    Carotid-cavernous fistula
    Carotid artery occlusive disease

ACUTE IRITIS VERSUS ACUTE GLAUCOMA

	Acute iritis	**Acute glaucoma**
Pressure	Decreased, normal or mildly elevated intra-ocular pressure	Rapid, severe elevation of intra-ocular pressure; hard globe
Anterior chamber depth	Normal	Shallow with iridocorneal contact and shallow contralateral anterior chamber with a narrow angle
Pupil	Small	Middilated and deformed
Injection	Ciliary injection	Limbal and conjunctival congested blood vessels
Cornea	Usually clear except for the presence of keratic precipitates	Oedema
History	Occasionally association with systemic diseases (e.g. ankylosing spondylitis, sarcoidosis); often history of ipsilateral previous attacks	Previous episodes of coloured haloes with transient blurring of vision and pain, which typically occurred in darkened conditions
Pain	Mild, dull pain of the involved eye	Acute onset of severe periocular pain
General condition	Usually normal	Unwell; the pain often radiates to the head, occasionally accompanied by nausea and vomitting

MEDICAL TREATMENT OF GLAUCOMA

Action profile of antiglaucomatous drugs

Increase of aqueous outflow		Decrease of aqueous production	
Parasympatho-mimetics	Adrenergic agonists	Carbonic anhydrase inhibitors	β-blockers
Pilocarpine	Dipivefrine	Acetazolamide	Timolol
Carbachol	Adrenaline		etc.

Drug	Onset	Maximal action	Duration
Pilocarpine	30 min	2 hours	8 hours
Beta-blocker	30 min	2 hours	24 hours
Dipivefrin	15–30 min	2 hours	8 hours
Latanoprost	3–4 hours	8–12 hours	24 hours
Acetazolamide			
• tablets	30–90 min	2 hours	6 hours
• SR capules		8 hours	12 hours
• intravenous		15 min	4 hours
Dorzolamide (topical)	30 min	2–3 hours	10 hours
Glycerol (oral)	10 min	30 min	3–5 hours
Mannitol 20% (intravenous over 30 min)	20–60 min		2–6 hours

MEDICAL TREATMENT OF GLAUCOMA

Parasympathomimetics (pilocarpine)	Heart failure Asthma Hyperthyroidism Gastric and duodenal ulcers Intestinal obstruction (ileus) Urinary retention
Sympathomimetics (dipivefrin)	Angle-closure glaucoma Phaeochromocytoma
Beta-blockers	Asthma Atrioventricular block (II°nd & III°) Decompensated heart failure Depression Keratoconjunctivitis sicca
Carbonic anhydrase inhibitors	Pregnancy Sulphonamide allergy Oliguria, anuria Kidney stones Loop diuretics Digitalis (e.g. digoxin) Acetylsalicylic acid Chronic lung disease (respiratory acidosis) Blood dyscrasias (thrombocytopenia, agranulocytosis and aplastic anaemia may occur as idiosyncratic reactions to carbonic anhydrase inhibitors)
Hyperosmotic agents	Congestive heart failure Oliguria, anuria Severe hypertension

ASPECTS IN THE CHOICE OF ANTIGLAUCOMATOUS DRUGS

Pigment dispersion glaucoma	As in primary open-angle glaucoma (initially β-blockers or sympathomimetics; topical acetazolamide or miotics if sufficient pressure reduction not achieved)
Plateau iris syndrome	Miotics
Glaucoma and lens opacity	Miotics undesirable
Raised episcleral venous pressure	Pilocarpine application may result in elevation of the episcleral venous pressure
Intraocular inflammation	Pilocarpine increases the permeability of the blood–aqueous humour barrier, which allows the transfer of proteins into the aqueous humour and increases the risk of posterior synechiae formation
Obstructive respiratory disease (except asthma)	Selective β_1-blocker (betaxolol) can be tried, whereas nonselective β-blockers are contra-indicated
Asthma	β-blocker contraindicated; pilocarpine may lead to increased bronchial secretion and bronchospasm
Kidney stones	Avoid carbonic anhydrase inhibitors

GLAUCOMA FOLLOW-UP

RECOMMENDATION FOR IOP CHECK-UP AFTER COMMENCEMENT OF TREATMENT

Beta-blockers
- Depending on initial IOP first check-up 3–4 weeks after commencement of treatment (ideally, only one eye should be treated initially to enable the contralateral eye to act as a control)
- Ideally, a 24-hour IOP should be done four weeks after commencement of treatment
- Three or six monthly IOP check-ups (depending on IOP, disc, visual field)

Parasympathomimetics
- As β-blockers
- In addition, unilateral one-drop assessment is sometimes performed: after topical application in one eye, the IOP is obtained (every half hour, later every hour) from both eyes, whereas in contact tonometry the nontreated eye is measured first

Dipivefrine
- As β-blockers

Decline of action

- Discontinue the drug
- Note prolonged action three days after stopping pilocarpine and up to one week after stopping adrenaline or β-blockers

Combined topical treatment

1. β-blocker and topical acetazolamide
2. β-blocker and pilocarpine
3. β-blocker and dipivefrine (usually avoided because of side-effects)
4. Guanethidine and dipivefrine
5. β-blocker, dipivefrine and acetazolamide derivative
6. Add oral acetazolamide if needed (short-term)

MANAGEMENT OF ACUTE ANGLE-CLOSURE GLAUCOMA

- Acetazolamide 500 mg i.v., then sustained-release acetazolamide 250 mg twice daily
- Topical β-blocker twice daily (if not contraindicated)
- Topical steroids four times daily
- In insufficient response, use hyperosmotic agents
- Approx 30 min after commencement of treatment: topical pilocarpine 2% every 15 min for one hour, then four times daily (at high pressure, the iris sphincter is ischaemic and unresponsive to pilocarpine)
- Topical pilocarpine 1% four times daily to the fellow eye
- If no response after six hours, consider laser iridotomy or peripheral iridectomy

- Once the corneal oedema resolves and the pressure is medically controlled, YAG laser iridotomy can be performed. Contralateral prophylactic YAG laser iridotomy can be carried out at the same session
- In cases of no compliance or if YAG laser is not available, consider peripheral iridectomy or filtration surgery

MANAGEMENT OF MALIGNANT GLAUCOMA

- Long-term daily mydriatic–cycloplegic drops (atropine 1% four times daily)
- Short-term acetazolamide 250 mg four times daily and infusion of hyperosmotic mannitol, 1–2 g per kg body weight (20% solution)
- If the medical treatment is unsatisfactory, surgical intervention should be considered (laser iridotomy, peripheral iridectomy, lens extraction)
- In aphakic eyes, consider vitreous aspiration

ARGON LASER TRABECULOPLASTY

ARGON LASER TRABECULOPLASTY (ALT)

(Wise JB, Witter SL (1979) Argon laser therapy for open angle glaucoma. *Arch Ophthalmol* **97**:319–322)

Indication	Open-angle to topical treatment glaucoma in patients with insufficient response or low compliance with the same, and following filtration surgery which did not achieve intraocular pressures within normal limits
Contra-indication	Invisibility of the trabeculum (e.g. closed or narrow angle, blood obscuring the angle, hazy cornea), paediatric glaucoma, secondary glaucoma, previously failed ALT
Extent	180°
Viewing power	The slit lamp is utilized with a gonioscopic lens with 25-fold ocular viewing power
Direction	The beam is to be focused at the junction between the pigmented and nonpigmented trabeculum
Spot size	50 µm
Duration	0.1 sec
Energy	700–1500 mW (aim is to achieve transient blanching or bubble formation at the point of impact). Note that less pigmented angles require higher energy
Number of burns	Approximately 100

PLACEMENT OF THE ARGON LASER BEAM FOCUS

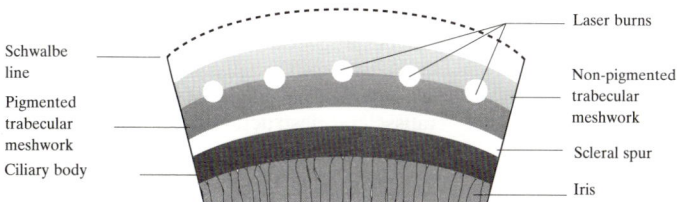

Schwalbe line — Laser burns — Pigmented trabecular meshwork — Non-pigmented trabecular meshwork — Ciliary body — Scleral spur — Iris

CYCLOCRYOTHERAPY

Indication	Glaucomatous eyes in which normal IOP could not be achieved with other measures
Probe diameter	2.5 mm
Placement	The edge of the probe is placed 1–1.5 mm from the limbus, so that the distance between the limbus and the centre of the burn is 3–4 mm
Number of burns	3–4 per quadrant (total of two quadrants)
Temperature	−60 to −80°C
Duration	60 sec per burn
Medical therapy	Initially the glaucomatous medical treatment is to be continued
Re-treatment	If sufficient reduction of pressure has not been achieved after 4 weeks, re-treat the same quadrants. The other half of the circumference is to be treated if the second treatment fails to achieve satisfactory results

GLAUCOMA SURGERY

FISTULIZING PROCEDURES

Trabeculectomy	Excision of a corneoscleral block with knife
Trephine operation	Block excision via a trephine
Filtration surgery with scleral flap	Excision of a deep limbal corneal block with knife or trephine under a partial-thickness scleral flap
Molteno tube	Insertion of a silicone tube in the anterior chamber
Iridokleisis	Incarceration of iris in a scleral incision after peripheral iridectomy

PROCEDURES INVOLVING IRIS, TRABECULAR MESHWORK OR CILIARY BODY

Peripheral iridectomy	Removal of peripheral iris
Laser iridotomy	Peripheral perforation of the iris with YAG laser
Argon laser trabeculoplasty	Photocoagulation of the trabecular meshwork
Goniotomy	Incision in the trabecular meshwork to establish communication between the anterior chamber and Schlemm's canal
Trabeculotomy (external goniotomy)	A trabeculotome is introduced through a scleral flap and into Schlemm's canal to establish communication to the anterior chamber
Cyclodialysis	Disinsertion of the ciliary body from the scleral spur
Cyclocryotherapy	Transscleral destruction of the ciliary processes at very low temperature
Transscleral cyclophotocoagulation	Destruction of ciliary body by YAG laser

IRIS DEFORMATIONS AND ANOMALIES

CONGENITAL AND ACQUIRED IRIS CHANGES

Corectopia (congenital)

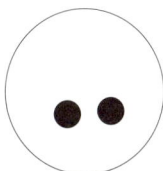

Polycoria (congenital)

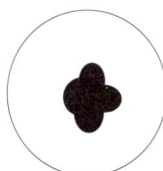

Iris bombe (due to circumferential posterior synechiae–seclusio pupillae)

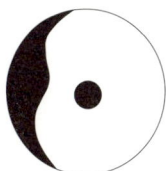

Iridodialysis with displaced pupil (posttraumatic)

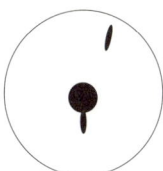

Iridotomy (after YAG laser treatment) and sphinctero-tomy (postoperative)

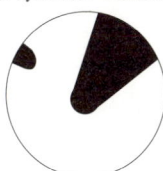

Peripheral iridectomy and sector iridectomy (postoperative)

CHARACTERISTICS OF THE IRIDOCORNEAL ENDOTHELIAL SYNDROMES (ICES)

Common features of the three ICES

- Corneal endothelial dystrophy
- Distorted pupil
- Ectropion uveae
- Goniosynechiae
- Secondary synechial glaucoma

Characteristics that distinguish between the three ICES

- Iris naevus syndrome (Cogan–Reese)
  Multiple small or a few larger iris nodules
- Chandler's syndrome
  Corneal oedema at normal or mildly elevated IOP
  Only mild or absent iris changes
- Essential iris atrophy
  Progressive iris atrophy with iris hole formation (opposite to the side of the goniosynechiae)

IRIDOCORNEAL DYSGENESIS

PERIPHERAL AND CENTRAL CONGENITAL CORNEAL MALFORMATIONS

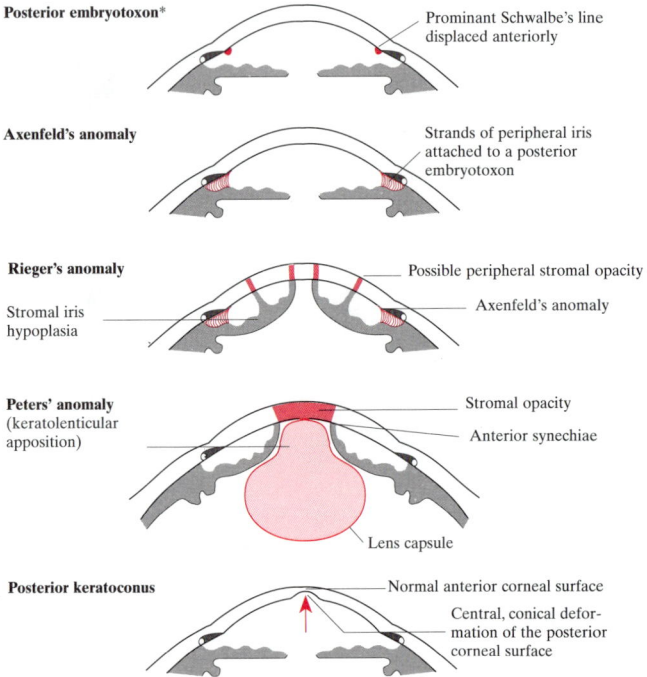

Posterior embryotoxon*

Prominant Schwalbe's line displaced anteriorly

Axenfeld's anomaly

Strands of peripheral iris attached to a posterior embryotoxon

Rieger's anomaly

Stromal iris hypoplasia

Possible peripheral stromal opacity

Axenfeld's anomaly

Peters' anomaly
(keratolenticular apposition)

Stromal opacity

Anterior synechiae

Lens capsule

Posterior keratoconus

Normal anterior corneal surface

Central, conical deformation of the posterior corneal surface

*The presence of a posterior embryotoxon indicates paediatric referral to exclude Alagille's syndrome (arteriohepatic dysplasia)

ICE SYNDROMES (COGAN–REESE, CHANDLER'S, ESSENTIAL IRIS ATROPHY) VERSUS IRIDOCORNEAL DYSGENESES (AXENFELD–RIEGER)

	ICE	Axenfeld–Rieger
Manifestation	Unilateral	Bilateral
Endothelium	Dystrophy	Normal
Angle	Goniosynechiae	Iris strands
Iris stroma	Abnormal	Abnormal
Ectropion uveae	Present	Present
Glaucoma	100% of cases	60% of cases
Age	20–30 years	Congenital
Sex	Mostly females	Males = females
Inheritance	Sporadic	Autosomal dominant

ANGLE TRAUMA IN BLUNT EYE INJURY

Angle trauma in blunt eye injury

Angle recession
Separation between the longitudinal and circular fibres of the ciliary muscle

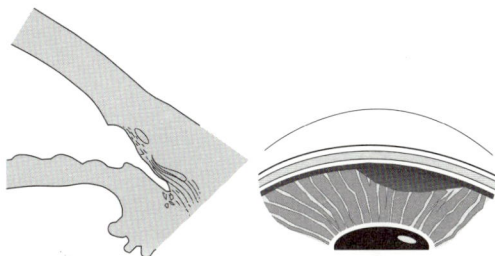

Cyclodialysis cleft
Disinsertion of the ciliary body from the scleral spur (allows free access of aqueous humour into the suprachoroidal space; and often results in decreased IOP)

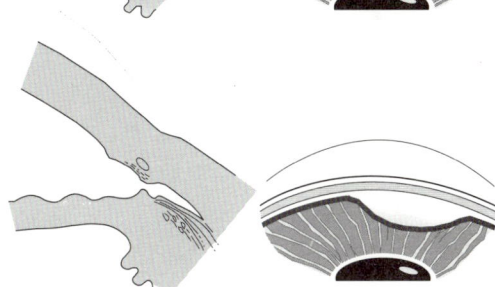

Iridodialysis
Tear through the peripheral iris (disinsertion of the iris root from the ciliary body)

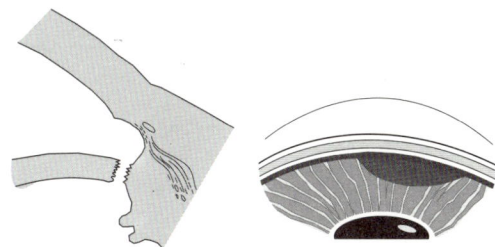

Trabecular injury
Tear in the anterior part of the trabecular meshwork

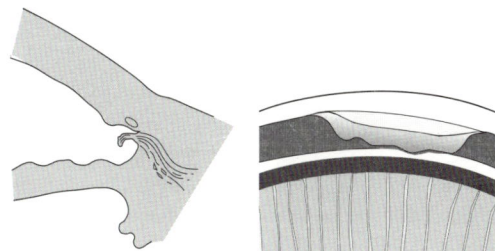

Chapter 7

LENS

CATARACT

CAUSES OF CATARACT

Senile cataract	Age-related lens opacity is the most common cause of cataracts
Congenital cataracts	• $^1/_3$ inherited • $^1/_3$ associated with other syndromes • $^1/_3$ idiopathic
Cataracts associated with systemic diseases	• Metabolic diseases (e.g. diabetes mellitus, galactosaemia, hypocalcaemia, Wilson's disease, Fabry's disease) • Dermatogenic (e.g. atopic dermatitis, vitiligo) • Nutritional deficiency (e.g. anorexia nervosa) • Myotonic dystrophy
Posttraumatic cataract	• Blunt eye injury • Perforating eye injury • Chemical injuries • Electrical injury
Radiation-induced cataracts	• Ionizing radiation • Infrared radiation (glassblowers' cataract) • Ultraviolet radiation
Drug-induced cataracts	• Corticosteroids • Phenothiazines • Miotics • Amiodarone
Cataracts associated with hereditary fundus dystrophies	e.g. retinitis pigmentosa, Stickler's syndrome, Leber's congenital amaurosis
Miscellaneous	e.g. chronic uveitis, high myopia

ANATOMY OF THE LENS

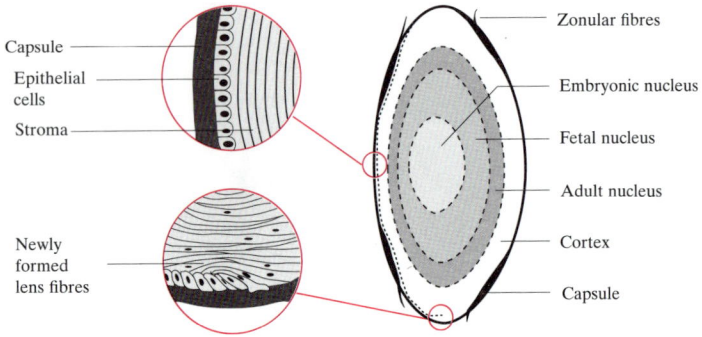

Capsule
Epithelial cells
Stroma

Newly formed lens fibres

Zonular fibres
Embryonic nucleus
Fetal nucleus
Adult nucleus
Cortex
Capsule

CLASSIFICATION OF CATARACTS

Appearance	Maturity	Cause
Membranous	Incipient	Senile
Subcapsular	Advanced	Secondary
Lamellar	Mature	Congenital
Stellate	Hypermature	Traumatic
Cortical	Morgagnian	Dermatogenic
Nuclear		Radiation-induced
Complete		Drug-induced
Intumescent		Miscellaneous
Brunescent		

MORPHOLOGICAL CLASSIFICATION OF CATARACT

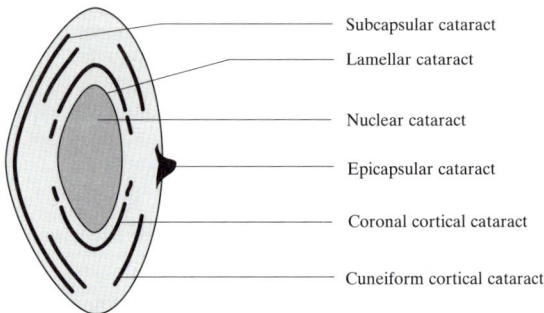

Subcapsular cataract
Lamellar cataract
Nuclear cataract
Epicapsular cataract
Coronal cortical cataract
Cuneiform cortical cataract

SECONDARY CATARACT

CATARACTOGENIC DRUGS

Corticosteroids
Systemic and topical application; subcapsular cataract

Phenothiazines
Pigmented deposits in the anterior suture pattern of the lens

Amiodarone
Cornea verticillata occurs on moderate to high daily doses; anterior subcapsular lens opacities may coexist

Cytostatics (e.g. busulphan)

A recognized but not common cause of cataract formation

Myotics
In particular, long-acting anticholinesterases

Metal-containing drugs
e.g. gold, mercury

LENS DISLOCATION

OCULAR CONDITIONS WHICH MAY BE ASSOCIATED WITH DISPLACEMENT OF THE LENS

Posttraumatic
Marfan's syndrome
High myopia
Idiopathic (ectopia lentis)
Corectopia
Buphthalmos (hydrophthalmos)
Megalocornea, cornea plana
Aniridia
Weill–Marchesani's syndrome
Homocystinuria
Hyperlysinaemia
Sulphite oxidase deficiency

Uveitis
Persistent hyperplastic primary vitreous humour (PHPV)
Ehlers–Danlos' syndrome
Scleroderma
Alport's syndrome
Mandibulofacial dysostosis
Klinefelter's syndrome
Renitis pigmentosa
Axenfeld–Rieger's syndrome
Crouzon's syndrome
Refsum's syndrome

CONGENITAL CATARACTS

DIFFERENTIAL DIAGNOSIS OF LEUKOCORIA IN CHILDREN

- Congenital cataract
- Persistent hyperplastic primary vitreous humour (PHPV)
- Tumours
    Retinoblastoma
    Medulloblastoma

- Retinal dysplasia (bilateral involvement in Norrie's disease and Patau's syndrome)
- Coats' disease
- Retinopathy of prematurity
- Toxocaral granuloma

Diagnosis	Age at presentation	Unilateral	Bilateral
Congenital cataract	Newborn		90%
Retinopathy of prematurity	Newborn		100%
Persistent hyperplastic primary vitreous humour	Newborn	90%	
Retinoblastoma	Up to 4 years		30%
Coats' disease	Usually in the first decade	80%	

THE VARIOUS PRESENTATIONS OF CONGENITAL CATARACT

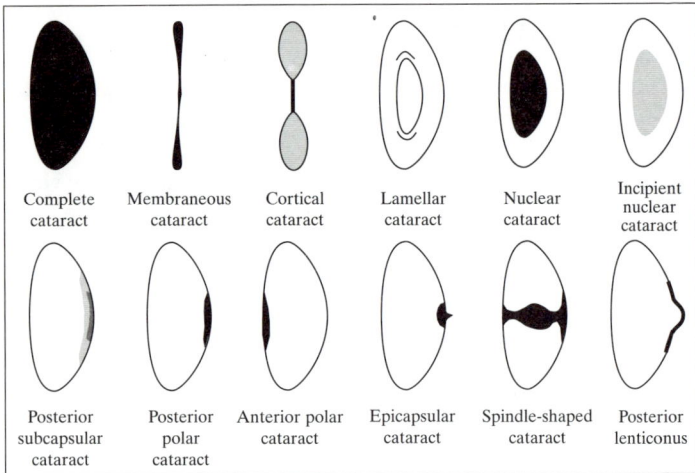

Complete cataract | Membraneous cataract | Cortical cataract | Lamellar cataract | Nuclear cataract | Incipient nuclear cataract

Posterior subcapsular cataract | Posterior polar cataract | Anterior polar cataract | Epicapsular cataract | Spindle-shaped cataract | Posterior lenticonus

CATARACT SURGERY

CONTRA-INDICATIONS TO CATARACT SURGERY

[O'Day DM and the Cataract Management Guideline Panel of the Agency for Health Care Policy and Research (1993) Management of cataract in adults. *Arch Ophthalmol* 111:453–459]

- The indication for cataract operation has been established, but the patient is not keen to undergo surgery
- Postoperative visual improvement is expected, but patient happy with current vision
- Postoperative improvement of lifestyle is not expected
- Surgery under local anaesthesia not possible but general anaesthesia is contra-indicated

INDICATIONS FOR CATARACT SURGERY UNDER GENERAL ANAESTHESIA

- Anxiety which does not allow surgery under local anaesthesia
- Insufficient communication between patient and surgeon (e.g. marked limited language difficulties, mental disability)
- Known allergy to local anaesthetic agents
- Conditions which cannot be sufficiently controlled during the operation (e.g. Parkinson's disease, marked low back pain)

THE INCIDENCE OF POSTOPERATIVE COMPLICATIONS IN STRAIGHTFORWARD CATARACT SURGERY

[Cataract Management Guideline Panel (1993) Management of functional impairment due to cataract in adults. *Ophthalmology* 100:41S]

≥1 in 100	Glaucoma, ptosis, haemorrhages, glare, cystoid macular oedema, allergic reaction to postoperative treatment (e.g. neomycin allergy)
1 in 100	Dislocated implant, mydriasis, endophthalmitis, retinal detachment, bullous keratopathy
1 in 1000	Depression, visual loss, diplopia
1 in 10000	Chronic pain, psychosis, expulsive haemorrhage
1 in 100000	Death, suicide

BIOMETRY

CALCULATION OF IOL POWER

SRK formula

[Sanders DR, Retzlaff J, Kraff MC (1983) Comparison of empirical derived and theoretical aphakic refraction formulas. *Arch Ophthalmol* 101:965–967]

$$D = A - 2.5L - 0.9K$$

D = Lens implant power for emmetropia (dpt)
A = Constant specific to the lens implant to be used (A-constant)
L = Axial length (mm)
K = Average keratometric reading (dpt)

Conversion of the original SRK formula to the SRK II formula

Short axial length (L less than 22 mm)

21–22 mm: add 1 dpt to the precalculated emmetropic power
20–21 mm: add 2 dpt to the precalculated emmetropic power
10–20 mm: add 3 dpt to the precalculated emmetropic power

Long axial length

L more than 24.5 mm: subtract 0.5 dpt from the precalculated emmetropic power

Source of errors in the calculation of the IOL power

Difference of 0.1 mm in the corneal radius   0.5 dpt
Difference of 0.1 mm in the axial length   0.3 dpt
Difference of 0.1 mm in the position of the implant 0.2 dpt

POSTOPERATIVE CARE

CRITERIA FOR DISCHARGE AFTER DAY CASE CATARACT SURGERY

• Patient happy to go home
• An escort to take the patient home is desirable
• Management of the postoperative care explained to the patient or to the escort
• Postoperative medication and written instructions for the post-operative care given
• Postoperative follow-up appointment made
• Availability of a 24 hour ophthalmic emergency service guaranteed

IDEAL POSTOPERATIVE FOLLOW-UP AFTER UNCOMPLICATED DAY CASE CATARACT SURGERY

[O'Day DM and the Cataract Management Guideline Panel of the Agency for Health Care Policy and Research (1993) Management of cataract in adults. *Arch Ophthalmol* 111:453–459]

Vision, IOP, biomicroscopy, consultation	1st postoperative day
	1st postoperative week
	3 weeks postoperatively
	6–8 weeks postoperatively
Fundoscopy	Once during the postoperative follow-ups
Refraction	6–12 weeks postoperatively (ECCE)

POSSIBLE COMPLICATIONS AFTER YAG LASER CAPSULOTOMY

- Raised intraocular pressure
- Damage to implant
- Hyphaema
- Corneal oedema
- Intraocular inflammation
- Cystoid macular oedema
- Retinal detachment

GOALS AND MANAGEMENT OF POST-OPERATIVE REFRACTIVE RESULT

- Emmetropia/myopia up to -3.0 dpt (a postoperative myopic outcome is preferred in patients with highly myopic preoperative refractive state)
- Consider the difference in the refractive error of the two eyes (in post-operative anisometropia, arrange for contralateral cataract surgery in the near future)
- Avoid postoperative aniseikonia

PHACO-EMULSIFICATION

WHY PHACO-EMULSIFICATION

Some surgeons argue that although there is an earlier visual recovery and an earlier return to full activity with smaller incisions of phaco-emulsification, by 4–8 weeks postoperatively there is no significant difference in the visual outcome among patients who have undergone uncomplicated extracapsular cataract extraction (ECCE) with conventional incision and patients who have had uncomplicated phaco-emulsification procedure with small incision.

However, there is growing evidence that in the hands of an experienced surgeon, phaco-emulsification is a quick and safe procedure (although a long learning curve usually precedes skilled technique), with a lower incidence of wound-related complications, reduced postoperative inflammation, minimal postoperative astigmatism and more rapid visual rehabilitation than found in large-incision procedures, all of which justify its higher costs.

Surgical technique

[Fischel JD, Lipton JR (1996) Clear-corneal incision length decreased to 2.5 mm. *Ocul Surg News* **14(15)**:20]

The surgery starts with a two-step stab incision at the superior limbus through the cornea. Sodium hyaluronate is used to fill the anterior chamber. Capsulorhexis is started by introducing an irrigating cystotome into the anterior chamber and making a small flap in the anterior capsule. The capsulorhexis is then completed with capsulorhexis forceps.

Hydro-dissection is performed with a hydro-dissector needle and balanced salt solution (BSS). Phaco-emulsification of the nucleus is completed a safe distance from the posterior capsule. Irrigation with aspiration of the cortex is performed once the nucleus has been removed. Sodium hyaluronate is then used to inflate the capsular bag and a one-piece foldable intraocular lens implant is injected into the posterior chamber using a cartridge and introducer. If the posterior capsule is not intact, a foldable three-piece lens is placed in the ciliary sulcus. The operation ends with a subconjunctival injection of mixed antibiotics and corticosteroids at the lower fornix. Foldable lenses are not always used in phaco-emulsification (due to expense).

Placement of the sutureless wound

In the presence of against-the-rule astigmatism, a temporal incision is used so that flattening of the steeper meridian with subsequent beneficial post-operative drift of astigmatism is achieved.

Note that operating through a temporal incision is technically more difficult, as the patient's forehead is not available to support the surgeon's wrist.

A combined phaco-emulsification and trabeculectomy procedure is always carried out at the superior limbus regardless of the preoperative astigmatism. In the presence of high against-the-rule astigmatism, a temporal transverse keratotomy may be added at the end of the procedure.

Intraoperative posterior capsule rupture

- Small holes in the posterior capsule are managed as follows:
  Anterior vitrectomy if needed;
  Sodium hyaluronate anterior to the anterior capsule;
  A foldable posterior chamber implant with footplates placed in the ciliary sulcus (the previously performed capsulorhexis should not have too large a diameter leaving sufficient anterior capsule support to secure the implant posteriorly);
  Irrigation/aspiration
- Small pieces of soft lens matter that fall into the vitreous humour may cause transient post-operative rise in the intraocular pressure, but usually no further problems.
- Large pieces of nucleus lost into the vitreous humour can be carefully chased with the anterior vitrectomy tip (but never with the phaco-emulsification probe).
- Lost lens matter or a dropped implant, once it has sunk to lie on the retina, should be left well alone. If removal is desired, the eye should be left aphakic and the patient referred to a vitreoretinal surgeon.
- Large posterior capsule ruptures and insufficient anterior capsule support for a sulcus-based lens require enlargement of the corneal incision to enable insertion of an anterior chamber implant with prophylactic peripheral iridectomy. Alternatively, placement of a scleral-sutured sulcus-fixated posterior chamber implant may be carried out.

Notes for the beginner

- Leave cases which are prone to zonule dialysis (e.g. pseudo-exfoliation syndrome) to high-volume phaco-emulsification surgeons.

- Dense cataract in the elderly typically presents with a hard nucleus; again leave to the experienced surgeon.
- If a second instrument is preferred, a second stab incision is made on the side of the surgeon's nondominant hand. It is placed $2\frac{1}{2}$–3 clock hours apart from the first incision for the 'divide and conquer' technique and $1\frac{1}{2}$–2 clock hours apart from the first incision for the 'chip and flip' technique.
- After cracking the nucleus, use suction forces ('follow-ability') to pick up nucleus particles with the tip of the phaco-emulsification probe. During the emulsification procedure, keep the particles at the pupillary plane to allow a safe distance from the posterior capsule on the one hand and the corneal endothelium on the other.
- Small pupils do not necessarily have to be stretched prior to surgery as long as the surgeon does not allow the phaco-emulsifier tip to come into contact with the iris and avoids using the phaco-emulisifier probe blindly behind the iris.

Chapter 8

UVEA

ANATOMY OF THE UVEAL TRACT

The uveal tract is a vascular pigmented layer which consists, from posterior to anterior, of the choroid, ciliary body and the iris.

Choroid	Ciliary body	Iris
Suprachoroid	Suprachoroid	Anterior epithelium
Stroma	Cilliary muscle	Dilator pupillae muscle
Choriocapillaris	Vessel layer	Stroma
Bruch's membrane	Basement membrane of the pigmented epithelium Outer pigmented epithelium Inner nonpigmented epithelium Basement membrane of the nonpigmented epithelium	Posterior epithelial layer

THE UVEAL BLOOD SUPPLY

Arterial supply
Anterior segment
- Two long posterior ciliary arteries
  Arise from the ophthalmic artery, pierce the sclera on the nasal and temporal sides of the optic nerve and run forward below the medial rectus and lateral rectus respectively
- Seven anterior ciliary arteries
  Arise from the muscular branches of the ophthalmic artery to the four recti (two arteries to each muscle, but only one artery to the lateral rectus)

Posterior segment
- 6–20 short posterior ciliary arteries
  Arise from the ophthalmic artery, pierce the sclera near the optic nerve to form the circle of Zinn

Venous drainage
- 4–6 vortex veins
  Received by the ophthalmic vein

Blood–aqueous humour barrier
- Ciliary vessels (fenestrated endothelium): zonulae occludentes of the non-pigmented ciliary epithelium
- Iris vessels (nonfenestrated endothelium)

Blood–retina barrier
- Retinal vessels (nonfenestrated endothelium)
- Choroidal vessels (fenestrated endothelium): zonulae occludentes of the retinal pigment epithelium

CLINICAL EVALUATION OF UVEITIS

ANATOMICAL CLASSIFICATION OF UVEITIS (RECOMMENDATIONS OF THE INTERNATIONAL UVEITIS STUDY GROUP)

[Bloch-Michel E, Nussenblatt RB (1978) International Uveitis Study Group recommendations for the evaluation of intraocular inflammatory disease. *Am J Ophthalmol* **103**:234]

Anterior uveitis	Iritis
Anterior cyclitis	Iridocyclitis
Intermediate uveitis	Previously known as pars planitis, posterior cyclitis, basal retinochoroiditis, peripheral uveitis
Posterior uveitis	Focal, multifocal or diffuse choroiditis, chorioretinitis
Panuveitis	

GRADING OF AQUEOUS CELLS

Cells	Grade	Tyndall phenomenon
<5	0	Clear aqueous humour
5–10	+1	Aqueous humour nearly clear
10–20	+2	Cells definitely identifiable
20–50	+3	Hazy iris details
>50	+4	Aqueous humour appears white

GRADING OF AQUEOUS FLARE

Flare	Grade	Tyndall phenomenon
Faint	+1	Aqueous humour nearly clear
Mild	+2	Clear iris details
Moderate	+3	Hazy iris details
Intense	+4	Aqueous humour with severe fibrinous exudate

CRITERIA FOR CLINICAL EVALUATION OF UVEITIS

Involvement	Iris, ciliary body, retina, choroid, blood vessels, complete inner eye
Extent	Focal, multifocal, diffuse
Appearance	Serous, fibrinous, granulomatous
Intensity	High, low
Manifestation	Sudden, gradual

Course   Simple, recurrent, chronic
Coexisting inflammation   Keratitis, scleritis, optic neuritis

DIFFERENTIAL DIAGNOSIS OF UVEITIS

IRIS FINDINGS IN ANTERIOR UVEITIS

Granuloma   Predominantly at the pupillary
                                          margin occurs in chronic
                                          inflammation such as:
                                          sarcoidosis
                                          syphilis
                                          tuberculosis
                                          Wegener's granulomatosis

Busacca nodules   Situated away from the pupillary
                                          margin, e.g. Vogt–Koyanagi–
                                          Harada syndrome

Koeppe nodules   Situated at the pupillary margin, e.g.
                                          sarcoidosis, tuberculosis

Atrophy (diffuse, focal, segmental)   Fuchs' heterochromic cyclitis, chronic
                                          iritis
                                          Herpes simplex iridocyclitis
                                          Herpes zoster iridocyclitis

Tumour   Haemangioma
                                          Malignant melanoma
                                          Metastases
                                          Infiltrating retinoblastoma
                                          Leukaemic infiltrates, malignant
                                          lymphoma
                                          Neurofibromatosis
                                          Juvenile xanthogranuloma

KERATIC PRECIPITATES (KP)

Morphology	Cellular deposits	Pathogenesis
Multiple fine, non-granulomatous precipitates	Predominantly leukocytes	**Acute iritis/iridocyclitis (e.g. juvenile rheumatoid arthritis, acute stage of chronic iridocyclitis)**
Few fine precipitates	Leukocytes	**Posner–Schlossman syndrome**
Multiple disseminated precipitates (also on the upper endothelium)	Leukocytes	**Fuchs' heterochromic cyclitis**

Morphology	Cellular deposits	Pathogenesis
Large granulomatous precipitates	Leukocytes, macrophages	**Chronic inflammation, sarcoidosis, tuberculosis** (practically never in HLA-B27 and associated anterior uveitis)

KEY FINDINGS OF INTERMEDIATE UVEITIS

- Anterior chamber shows no or minimal involvement
- Peripheral retinitis
- Perivasculitis
- Vitritis ('snowbanking', particularly in the inferior periphery)

INVESTIGATIONS IN UVEITIS

INDICATIONS FOR LABORATORY AND RADIOGRAPHIC INVESTIGATIONS IN ANTERIOR UVEITIS

Investigation	Indication for use
Serum angiotensin-converting enzyme (ACE)	Usually elevated in active systemic sarcoidosis (nonspecific)
Antinuclear antibodies (ANA)	Suspected Sjögren's syndrome, systemic lupus erythematosus, girls with oligoarthritis
Differential blood count	Regular monitoring in systemic steroid therapy, cytotoxic therapy
Lyme titre (*Borrelia burgdorferi*)	Uveitis with erythema migrans, history of tick bite, arthritis, neurological involvement (meningitis, cephalgia)
Epstein–Barr virus titre	Chronic bilateral iridocyclitis of unexplained origin
Fluorescent treponemal antibody absorption test	Suspected syphilis
Gallium scan	May be useful in suspected sarcoidosis (nonspecific, expensive)
HLA-B27	Acute unilateral iritis/iridocyclitis
Sacro-iliac X-ray	Suspected ankylosing spondylitis (pain in the sacroiliac region especially at night)
Rheumatoid factor (RF)	Not indicated
Chest X-ray	Suspected sarcoidosis, tuberculosis
Tine test and Heaf's test	To be done with chest X-rays when a positive history of tuberculosis is obtained; also indicated in chronic uveitis which deteriorates with steroid treatment

DIFFERENTIAL DIAGNOSIS OF INTERMEDIATE UVEITIS

Intraocular inflammations
Sarcoidosis
Chronic iridocyclitis
Vasculitis
Toxocariasis
Peripheral toxoplasmosis
CMV (cytomegalovirus) retinitis
Syphilis
Tuberculosis
Uveitis in multiple sclerosis

Other diseases
Retinoblastoma
Eales disease
Pars plana cysts
Sickle cell retinopathy
Equatorial retinal degenerations

ANTERIOR UVEITIS

HISTORY AND CLINICAL FINDINGS IN ANTERIOR UVEITIS

Finding/symptom	Aetiology	Further investigations
Arthritis	Ankylosing spondylitis	Sacroiliac X-rays, HLA-B27
	Behçet's disease	Fluorescein angiography, HLA-B5, dermatology
	Lyme disease	*Borrelia* titre
	Juvenile rheumatoid arthritis	Refer to paediatrician; antinuclear antibody, erythrocyte sedimeutation rate, HLA-B27
	Crohn's disease	Colonoscopy, HLA-B27
	Whipple's disease	Jejunum biopsy
	Psoriatic arthritis	Hand X-rays, HLA-B27
	Reiter's syndrome	Sacroiliac X-rays, HLA-B27
	Sarcoidosis	Chest X-rays, ACE, serum calcium level
Haemorrhagic enteritis	*Yersinia/Klebsiella enteritis*	Stool evaluation
	Sarcoidosis	Chest X-rays, ACE
Cephalgia	Sarcoidosis, Lyme disease (borrelia disease)	Chest X-rays, ACE, *Borrelia* titre
	Herpes zoster	Anti-viral antibodies
	Vogt–Koyanagi–Harada syndrome	Neurological referral
Haemorrhagic diathesis	Crohn's disease	Colonoscopy, HLA-B27
	Whipple's disease	Jejunum biopsy
	Yersinia/Klebsiella enteritis	Stool evaluation

Finding/symptom	Aetiology	Further investigations
Erythema nodosum	Crohn's disease	Colonoscopy, HLA-B27
	Psoriatic arthritis	Hand X-rays, HLA-B27
	Systemic lupus erythematosus	Antinuclear antibody, complement, medical referral
	Sarcoidosis	Chest X-rays, ACE
Erythema migrans	Lyme disease (borrelia disease)	*Borrelia* titre
Genital ulceration	Reiter's syndrome, Behçet's disease	Dermatology, fluorescein angiography, HLA-B5
Cough, dyspnoea	Sarcoidosis	Chest X-rays, ACE
	Tuberculosis	Chest X-rays, tine test, Heaf's test
	Neoplasm, metastases	Chest X-rays, medical referral
Oral ulceration	Behçet's disease	Fluorescein angiography, HLA-B5, dermatology
Parotid enlargement, lymphadenopathy	Sarcoidosis	Chest X-rays, ACE
Xerostomia (dry mouth)	Sjögren's syndrome	Antinuclear antibody, HLA-B27, medical opinion

HLA-B27-POSITIVE IRIDOCYCLITIS

OCCURRENCE AND INCIDENCE OF IMMUNOPATHOLOGICAL FEATURES

	HLA-B27	Rheumatoid factor	Antinuclear antibodies
General population	6%	3% (over 60 years of age: 10%)	5–10%
Acute anterior uveitis	60%		
Ankylosing spondylitis	95%		
Reiter's syndrome	70%	<10%	
Psoriatic arthritis			
without spinal involvement	25%		
with spinal involvement	60%		
Juvenile rheumatoid arthritis*	40%	10–20%	
Rheumatoid arthritis		80%	20%
Sjögren's syndrome		90%	75%
Systemic lupus erythematosus		25%	99%

*Approximately 30% of girls who are ANA+, HLA-B27− and RF− develop iridocyclitis. Boys who are HLA-B27+, ANA− and RF− often develop ankylosing spondylitis later in life

HLA-B27-POSITIVE ACUTE IRIDOCYCLITIS VERSUS HLA-B27-NEGATIVE ACUTE IRIDOCYCLITIS

[Rothava A *et al.* (1987) Clinical features of acute anterior uveitis. *Am J Ophthalmol* **103**:137–145]

	HLA-B27+	HLA-B27−
Average age (years)	35	43
Sex (M:F)	2.5:1	1:1
Bilateral onset	3%	21%
Alternating	38%	8%
Fibrin exudation	>50%	10%
Cells (+++) in AC	60%	20%
Vitreous cells (++)	55%	20%
Interval between attacks	~2 years	~1 year
Secondary manifestations		
Persistent posterior synechiae	36%	15%
Cataract	14%	6%
Glaucoma	8%	2%
Cystoid macular oedema	4%	−
Systemic disease		
Ankylosing spondylitis	39%	1%
Reiter's syndrome	8%	−
Psoriatic arthritis	4%	−
Syphilis	3%	7%

SPECIFIC UVEITIS SYNDROMES

IDIOPATHIC SPECIFIC UVEITIS SYNDROMES

	Acute posterior multifocal placoid pigment epitheliopathy (APMPPE)	Serpiginous choroiditis, geographic peripapillary choroiditis	Multi-focal choroiditis with panuveitis	Punctuate inner choroidopathy	Multiple evanescent white dot syndrome	Birdshot chorioretinitis
Age (years)	20–40	30–50	20–50	20–40	15–50	40–60
Sex	M = F	M = F	M < F	F (young, myopic)	F < M	M < F
Vitreous infiltration	Slight	Slight	Mild	None	Slight	Mild
Lesions	Grey/white	Geographic	Grey/white	Yellow/grey	Grey/white	Yellow/white
Macula	CNVM* rare	CNVM 25%	Central macular oedema, CNVM 35%	Atrophic scarring, CNVM 40%	CNVM rare	Yellow scarring, CNVM occasionally
Visual prognosis	Good	Poor	Good	Good	Good	Good

	Acute posterior multi-focal placoid pigment epitheliopathy (APMPPE)	Serpiginous choroiditis, geographic peripapillary choroiditis	Multi-focal choroiditis with panuveitis	Punctuate inner choroidopathy	Multiple evanescent white dot syndrome	Birdshot chorioretinitis
Associated HLA	B7, DR2	B7	?	?	?	A29
Therapy	Usually none	Steroids	Steroids	None	Steroids	Steroids

* Choroidal neovascular membrane

INTRAOCULAR INFLAMMATION WITH NEUROLOGICAL INVOLVEMENT

Multiple sclerosis — Periphlebitis
Vogt–Koyanagi–Harada syndrome — Meningoencephalitis
Behçet's disease — Meningoencephalitis
Sarcoidosis — Various manifestations
Reticulum cell sarcoma — Oculocerebral manifestation possible
Tertiary syphilis — Neurosyphilis, tabes dorsalis
Systemic lupus erythematosus — Paresis in 25% of cases, various symptoms
Wegener's granulomatosis — CNS granuloma, vasculitis, neuropathy
Herpes simplex — Meningitis
Congenital toxoplasmosis — Various manifestations
AIDS — Opportunistic infections with CNS involvement

TOXOPLASMIC RETINOCHOROIDITIS

SEROLOGICAL TESTS IN SUSPECTED TOXOPLASMIC RETINOCHOROIDITIS

Note:
- IgM and IgG tests are not necessarily positive in active toxoplasmic retinochoroiditis
- There is no serological test pronding a titre level that correlates with the probability or severity of toxoplasmic retinochoroiditis
- Results of antibody tests may not be correct if the patient's immune status is abnormal (e.g. in AIDS patients)

SCREENING TESTS FOR PREVIOUS TOXOPLASMOSIS INFECTION

Vitreous titre for complement binding reaction	$\geqslant 1:1$	Toxoplasmosis likely in a matching clinical picture
Indirect immunofluorescent antibody test		
Sabin–Feldman test		
Haemagglutination test	Positive	Toxoplasmosis likely

Indirect immunofluorescent antibody test Sabin–Feldman test	$\geqslant 1:256$	Inactive infection
Indirect immunofluorescent antibody test Sabin–Feldman test	$\geqslant 1:4096$	Active infection

TREATMENT OF TOXOPLASMIC RETINOCHOROIDITIS

Pyrimethamine triple therapy

Pyrimethamine	100 mg on the first day, then 25 mg daily for 3–4 weeks
	Contraindications:
	    pregnancy
	    severe blood disorders

Sulphadiazine	0.5–1 g four times daily
	Contraindications:
	    pregnancy
	    sulphadiazine allergy
	    renal failure
	    liver damage

Corticosteroids	60–100 mg prednisolone daily from 3rd–7th day after commencement of treatment, then taper off according to symptoms
Folic acid	3 mg twice weekly (prophylaxis of thrombocytopenia)

Clindamycin triple therapy

Clindamycin	150–300 mg four times daily as an alternative to pyrimethamine
	Further treatment as above
	Contraindications:
	    lincomycin hypersensitivity
	    severe intestinal disease (e.g. Crohn's disease)
	    caution if myasthenia gravis

SEROLOGICAL TESTS IN SUSPECTED SYPHILIS

SYPHILIS SCREENING

Intraocular inflammation indicates syphilis screening, because:

- the patient is asymptomatic between the syphilitic stages

- the right diagnosis may save the patient's life
- syphilis shows various ocular manifestations

Treponema pallidum haemagglutination (TPHA) test (syphilis screening)

High specificity; may be false-negative in the first 2–3 weeks after infection.

Fluorescent treponemal antibody absorption (FTA-Abs) test (confirmation of diagnosis)

If both TPHA and FTA-Abs are positive, the diagnosis of syphilis is considered proven.

Active/inactive syphilis?

Positive TPHA and FTA-Abs do not differentiate between active syphilis (requires treatment) and inactive syphilis. The following tests are used to confirm active syphilis:

1. Venereal Disease Research Laboratories (VDRL) test
2. IgM antibodies (ELISA, IgM-FTA-Abs, 19-S-IgM-FTA-Abs): IgM antibodies reach their peak level in the primary stage

Congenital syphilis

As IgM antibodies (in contrast to IgG antibodies) do not pass the placental barrier, their presence confirms congenital syphilis.

OCULAR INVOLVEMENT IN AIDS

Microangiopathy syndrome	Cotton wool spots (usually no specific treatment required as asymptomatic)
Opportunist infections	Cytomegaloretinitis (CMV retinitis) Toxoplasmic retinochoroiditis Acute retinal necrosis (herpes simpler virus, cytomegalovirus) is usually seen in patients who are otherwise well. Progressive outer retinal necrosis Fungal infections Syphilis Endogenous bacterial retinitis Pneumocystis carinii choroiditis

Neoplasmas	Kaposi's sarcoma (specific therapy usually not needed; other sarcomas may coincide)
Neuro-ophthalmological lesions	Motility disorders Pupillary disorders Cerebral toxoplasmosis Optic neuritis (rare)

GANCICLOVIR TREATMENT IN CMV RETINITIS

Mechanism of action	Inhibition of DNA polymerase
Application	Intravenous, intravitreal
Response	70–80% initial improvement 40–50% subsequent relapse
Side-effects	Myelosuppression
Initial treatment	5 mg per kg body weight twice daily (15–30 days)
Subsequent treatment	6 mg per kg body weight five times weekly or 10 mg per kg body weight three times weekly (not to be discontinued in AIDS patients as CMV retinitis is usually a preterminal sign)
Survival rate	8.5 months on average

LYME DISEASE

CLINICAL STAGES OF LYME DISEASE

Stage	Manifestation	Ocular involvement
Stage I (infection)	Erythema migrans Flu-like symptoms: elevated body temperature, lymphadenopathy Cephalgia Nausea Meningismus	Haemorrhagic conjunctivitis
Stage II (dissemination)	Chronic erythema migrans Myocarditis, arrhythmia Arthralgia (large joints) Hepatosplenomegalia Meningitis, encephalitis	Intraocular inflammation (various forms) Keratitis Pupillary abnormalities Extraocular muscle paresis
Stage III (organ manifestation, chronic inflammation)	Arthritis Myocarditis, pericarditis Encephalomyelitis Demyelinization Polyneuritis Dementia	As stage II

In an endemic region

History of a tick bite with erythema migrans within 3–30 days after exposure, or positive Lyme (*Borrelia*) titre with clinical involvement of at least one organ

In nonendemic region

Erythema migrans with positive Lyme titre, or erythema migrans with involvement of two or more organs (neurological/cardiac manifestations)

BACTERIAL ENDOPHTHALMITIS

Bacterial endophthalmitis

Course	Treatment
Infection without posterior segment involvement (**initial antibiotic treatment**)	**Topical** application: Antibiotic eye drops (e.g. gentamicin hourly) Mydriasis: atropine 1% eye drops twice daily **Sub-Tenon's** injection: e.g. gentamicin, vancomycin daily or every other day for approximately one week **Systemic** application: e.g. cefozalin (imipenem/cilastatin sodium)
Positive bacterial cultures allow coadministration of **steroids** (2–3 days after commencement of antibiotic treatment)	**Sub-Tenon's** steroid injection: dexamethasone 4 mg daily or every other day for approximately one week **Systemic** steroid therapy: prednisolone 40–80 mg daily in the morning for one or two weeks Note: in suspected **fungal** infection, steroids are contraindicated
Application of **intraocular therapy** is indicated if no improvement is achieved with the above treatment. In severe cases, **intravitreal** injection may be part of the initial treatment and is performed at the time of vitreous biopsy. An anterior chamber tap should be done.	e.g. gentamicin, cefazolin and dexamethasone, or tobramycin, cefazolin and dexamethasone, or gentamicin, vancomycin and dexamethasone, or amikacin, vancomycin and dexamethasone

- If the visual acuity deteriorates to perception of light within 24 hours after commencement of maximal therapy
- If there is no fundus view
- If ultrasonography indicates advanced diffuse vitreal involvement, vitreal abscess or tractions
- In endophthalmitis after surgical repair of a perforated eye injury
- In suspected fungal infection
- In infections with highly virulent organisms such as *Staphylococcus aureus*

MASQUERADE SYNDROMES

ANTERIOR SEGMENTS

	Age	Inflammation signs	Investigation
Retinoblastoma	<15 years	Vitreous infiltrates, cells, pseudohypopyon	Cytogenetics, calcifications on ultrasound and CT
Leukaemia	<15 years	Vitreous infiltrates, cells, heterochromia	Differential blood count, bone marrow biopsy, acqueous humour cytology
Intraocular foreign body	Any age	Vitreous infiltrates, cells	Radiographs of orbit, CT, ultrasound
Malignant melanoma	Any age	Vitreous infiltrates, cells	Red-free photography, ultrasound
Juvenile xanthogranuloma	<15 years	Cells in the anterior chamber, spontaneous hyphaema	Dermatological opinion, iris biopsy (response to steroid therapy)
Peripheral retinal detachment	Any age	Cells in the vitreous and anterior chamber	Ophthalmoscopy

POSTERIOR SEGMENTS

	Age	Inflammation signs	Investigation
Retinitis pigmentosa	Middle age, but may occur at any age	Vitreous infiltrates	ERG, EOG, visual fields

	Age	Inflammation signs	Investigation
Reticulum cell sarcoma	>35 years	Vitreous infiltrates, retinal exudates and haemorrhages, retinal pigment epithelium infiltrates, panuveitis	Diagnostic vitrectomy (cytology), aqueous humour cytology, cranial CT, MRI
Lymphoma	>15 years	Cotton wool spots, vasculitis, vitreous infiltrates, papilloedema, panuveitis	Lymph node biopsy, bone marrow puncture, medical referral, diagnostic vitrectomy (cytology)
Retinoblastoma	<5 years	Vitreous infiltrates, retinal exudates	Cytogenetics, calcifications on ultrasound and CT
Malignant melanoma	>15 years	Vitreous infiltrates	Red-free photography, ultrasound
Multiple sclerosis	>15 years	Periphlebitis	Neurological evaluation

CHOROIDAL DYSTROPHIES

CHORIOCAPILLARIS ATROPHY

- Central areolar choroidal dystrophy
- Peripapilliary choroidal atrophy
- Perimacular (anular) choroidal atrophy
- Diffuse choroidal atrophy

CHOROIDAL ATROPHY WITH INVOLVEMENT OF ALL THE CHOROIDAL LAYERS

- Central choroidal atrophy, high myopia
- Progressive bifocal choroidal atrophy; first temporal, then nasal (autosomal dominant)
- Peripapilliary choroidal atrophy
- Gyrate atrophy
- Diffuse choroidal atrophy, choroideremia (X-linked)

OCCURRENCE OF ANGIOID STREAKS

- Idiopathic
- Pseudoxanthoma elasticum
- Ehlers–Danlos syndrome

- Paget's disease
- Sickle cell anaemia
- Acromegalia
- Hypertension

CAUSES OF UVEAL EFFUSION (CHOROIDAL DETACHMENT)

Inflammatory	Trauma, intraocular surgery
	Scleritis, infected scleral buckling
	Cryocoagulation, photocoagulation
	Chronic uveitis, Vogt–Koyanagi–Harada syndrome
	Sympathetic ophthalmitis
Hydrostatic	Dural arteriovenous fistula
	Hypotension, penetrating wound
	Abnormal scleral thickness:
	anophthalmos
	emmetropia, myopia
	in association with Hunter's syndrome
Idiopathic	

TUMOURS OF THE UVEA

SYNOPSIS OF UVEAL TUMOURS

Neuro-epithelial tumours

- Leiomyoma (leiomyosarcoma) of the iris
- Medulloepithelioma
- Adenoma, adenocarcinoma of the pigmented or non-pigmented ciliary epithelium (rare)
- Pseudoadenomatous hyperplasia of the non-pigmented ciliary epithelium

Neuro-ectodermal tumours

- Neurilemmoma (Schwannoma), potentially malignant
- Neurofibroma
- Melanocytic naevus
- Malignant melanoma

Mesenchymal tumours

- Haemangioma of the iris and ciliary body
- Choroidal haemangioma
- Choroidal osteoma
- Xanthogranuloma
- Reticulum cell sarcoma

Metastases and leukaemia

NEURO-EPITHELIAL TUMOURS OF THE CILIARY BODY

[Zimmermann LE, Sobin LH (1980) Histological typing of tumors of the eye and its adnexa. International Histological Classification of Tumors. No 24. World Health Organization, Geneva]

I. Congenital tumours of the non-pigmented ciliary epithelium

A. Glioneuroma
B. Nonteratoid medulloepithelioma
C. Teratoid medulloepithelioma

II. Acquired tumours of the non-pigmented ciliary epithelium

A. Pseudoadenomatous hyperplasia
  • reactive hyperplasia
  • senile hyperplasia
B. Adenoma (solid, papilliary, pleomorphic)
C. Adenocarcinoma (malignant epithelioma) (solid, papilliary, pleomorphic)

III. Acquired tumours of the pigmented ciliary epithelium

Benign (adenoma)
Malignant (adenocarcinoma)

IV. Mixed tumours of the pigmented and nonpigmented ciliary epithelium

CHOROIDAL MELANOMA: CLINICAL FEATURES AND CLASSIFICATION

TYPICAL APPEARANCE OF MALIGNANT CHOROIDAL MELANOMA

• Accumulation of orange pigment (lipofuscin deposition)
• Large blood vessels clearly visible in amelanotic tumours
• A secondary exudative detachment, most commonly in the lower periphery, may develop
• A characteristic mushroom-shaped form develops as the tumour breaks through Bruch's membrane

ULTRASONOGRAPHY CHARACTERISTICS OF INTRA-OCULAR MELANOMA

• Choroidal excavation (echo-free zone at the tumour base)
• Orbital shadowing
• Often coexisting inferior retinal detachment

HISTOPATHOLOGICAL PROGNOSTIC FACTORS

Size   Larger tumours have a worse prognosis
Location   Disseminated infiltration of the choroid, involvement of the
                      anterior uveal segment and ciliary body, and extra-
                      ocular extension worsen the prognosis
Cell type   Spindle-A tumours have the best prognosis, epithelioid cell
                      tumours the worst
Mitosis activity A high mitosis rate worsens the prognosis
Pigmentation   Highly pigmented tumours have the worst prognosis,
                      amelanotic tumours the best

CYTOLOGICAL CLASSIFICATION OF MALIGNANT CHOROIDAL MELANOMA (WHO COMMISSION, 1979)

I. Spindle-cell type melanoma

1. 'Spindle A cell type' melanomas are composed of more than 75% spindle A cells. The rest of the cells are spindle B cells.
2. 'Spindle B cell type' melanomas are composed of more than 25% spindle B cells. The rest of the cells are predominantly spindle A cells with a minority of epithelioid cells.

II. Epithelioid cell melanoma

Composed of more than 75% epithelioid cells. The remainder are spindle A cells and/or spindle B cells

III. Mixed-cell melanoma (spindle and epithelioid cells)

1. Mixed-cell malignant melanoma with a dominance of spindle cells (but less than 75%)
2. Mixed-cell malignant melanoma with equally balanced spindle/epithelioid cells
3. Mixed-cell malignant melanoma with a dominance of epithelioid cells (but fewer than 75%)

IV. Others

All others are melanocytic malignant tumours that do not fit into the above criteria

TNM CLASSIFICATION FOR CHOROIDAL MELANOMA

T   **Primary tumour**. The tumour base is measured in papillary diameter (1 PD = 1.5 mm), the tumour height in dioptres (3 dpt = 1 mm). Ultrasound measurement is more precise
T0   No primary tumour
T1   Largest diameter of tumour base < 10 mm and tumour height <3 mm

T1a	Largest diameter of tumour base < 7 mm or tumour height < 2 mm
T1b	Largest diameter of tumour base > 7 mm but < 10 mm or tumour height > 2 mm but < 3 mm
T2	Largest diameter of tumour base > 10 mm but < 15 mm or tumour height > 3 mm but < 5 mm
T3	Largest diameter of tumour base > 15 mm or tumour height >5 mm
T4	Tumour with extraocular extension
TX	The extension of the primary tumour cannot be obtained
N	**Regional lymph node involvement**
N0	No involvement of regional lymph nodes
N1	Regional lymph nodes involved
NX	Examination of regional lymph nodes not possible
M	**Metastases**
M0	No metastases
M1	Evidence of metastases
MX	Screening for metastases cannot be undertaken
G	**Histopathological classification**
G1	Spindle-cell melanoma
G2	Mixed-cell melanoma
G3	Epithelioid cell melanoma
GX	Classification cannot be undertaken
S	**Scleral invasion**
S0	No scleral invasion
S1	Intrascleral invasion
S2	Extrascleral tumour
SX	Examination for scleral invasion cannot be undertaken
V	**Venous invasion**
V0	No venous invasion
V1	Melanoma veins contain tumour cells
VX	Venous invasion cannot be proven
pTMN	**Histopathological classification after enucleation**

DIFFERENTIAL DIAGNOSIS OF CHOROIDAL MELANOMA

Choroidal melanoma	Usually unilateral; fairly well-defined borders; most cases show elevation; occasionally amelanotic; often with superficial orange pigment and mushroom-shaped form as the tumour breaks through Bruch's membrane; exudative retinal detachment in the lower periphery
Choroidal naevus	Flat greyish, fairly well-defined lesion; no neoplastic hypervascularization (fluorescein angiography)
Choroidal metastases	Creamy yellow lesion with minimal elevation; ill-defined borders

Primary tumour is most commonly breast carcinoma (women) or bronchial carcinoma (men); other primary sites are gastrointestinal tumours, prostate carcinoma and others; one-third of all choroidal metastases are multifocal or bilateral (choroidal melanoma are unilateral in most cases).

Choroidal haemangioma

Deep red-orange, minimally elevated diffuse or circumscribed lesion
Secondary exudative retinal detachment
Hyperfluorescence in early stages
Peak prevalence at the age of 20–40 years
Diffuse choroidal haemangiomata sometimes occur in association with Sturge–Weber syndrome

RPE hyperplasia

Black pigmented, well-defined flat lesion; occasionally with central depigmentation; usually asymptomatic (unless the macula is involved); most commonly due to preceding trauma or inflammation, but may be associated with familial adenomatous polyposis

Melanocytoma

Usually inferior optic disc manifestation
Deep dark pigmentation of the superficial retinal layers, obscuring the underlying retinal vessels
More common in subjects with dark skin pigmentation

Choroidal osteoma

Rare. Women more often affected than men
Yellow white colour
Usually juxtapapillarily located
Bony plaque demonstrable with ultrasound or CT

Pseudotumours

Subretinal haemorrhages, choroidal detachment, macular degeneration, neovascular membranes, peripheral exudative retinal disorders, scleritis

Chapter 9

RETINA

LAYERS OF THE RETINA

Layers of the retina

I Pigment epithelium	A single layer of cuboidal cells
II Photoreceptors	Outer and inner segments of the rod and cone cells
III Outer limiting membrane	Radial processes of Müller cells
IV Outer nuclear layer	The nuclei of the rod and cone cells
V Outer plexiform layer	Synapses between the photoreceptor cells, the bipolar cells and the horizontal cells
VI Inner nuclear layer	Nuclei of the bipolar cells, the horizontal cells, the amacrine cells and the Müller cells
VII Inner plexiform layer	Synapses between the bipolar cells, amarcrine cells and ganglion cells
VIII Ganglion cell layer	Nuclei of the ganglion cells
XI Nerve fibre layer	Axons of the ganglion cells that merge together to build up the optic nerve
X Inner limiting membrane	Müller cell terminations and basement membrane

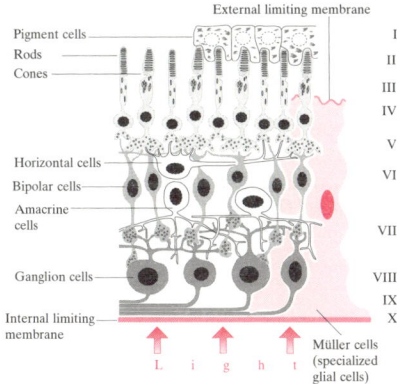

MACULA LUTEA AND FOVEA CENTRALIS

	Diameter
Macula	5.5 mm
Fovea	1.8 mm
Foveola	350 μm
Avascular zone	450 μm

Ratio macula : fovea : foveola = 16 : 5 : 1

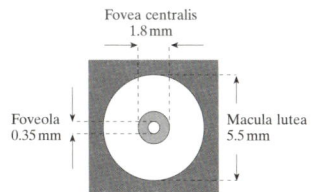

FUNDUS DIAGRAMS

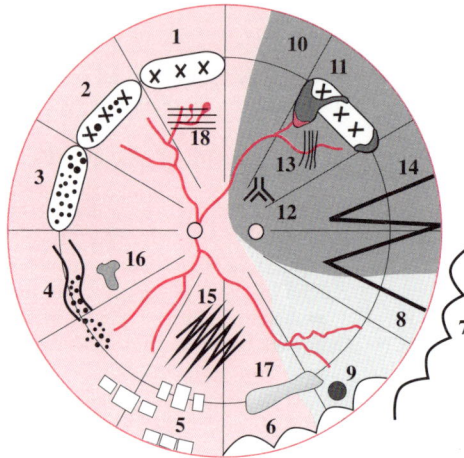

1. Lattice degeneration
2. Lattice degeneration, snowflakes and a small round hole
3. Snowflakes
4. Snailtrack and lattice degeneration
5. Paving stone degeneration
6. Ora serrata, visible without scleral indentation
7. Ora serrata visible with indentation
8. Shallow retinal detachment (light blue)
9. Equatorial round hole
10. Bullous retinal detachment
11. Horseshoe tear with equatorial degeneration
12. Star-shaped retinal folds
13. Vitreoretinal attachment
14. Cataract (reduced view)
15. Vitreous haemorrhage
16. Hyperpigmentation
17. Postoperative chorioretinal scarring
18. Neovascularization extending into the vitreous humour

Red	Attached retina, choroid, retinal arteries, haemorrhages
Blue	Detached retina, retinal veins, oedema, retinoblastoma
Blue hatchings	Lattice degeneration
Green	Fresh coagulation burns, vitreous opacities
Brown	Pigmented coagulation scars, melanoma, haemagioma, naevus
Yellow	Retinal exudates
Black	Retinal pigmentation

POSTOPERATIVE DOCUMENTATION

(may be added as planned procedure to the preoperative diagram)

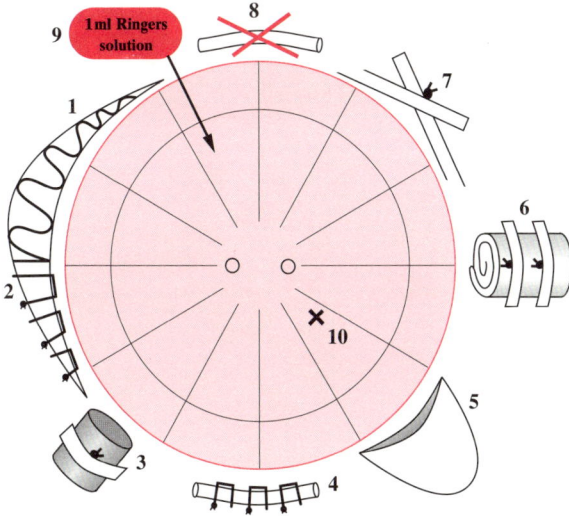

1. Scleral buckling
2. Lamellar scleral resection
3. Radial episcleral sponge seal
4. Segmental circumferential
   silicone sponge seal
5. Intrascleral cavity

6. Dural radial seal
7. Encircling circumferential seal
8. Removed seal
9. Intravitreal injection
10. Site of subretinal fluid drainage

POSTOPERATIVE FUNDUS DIAGRAM

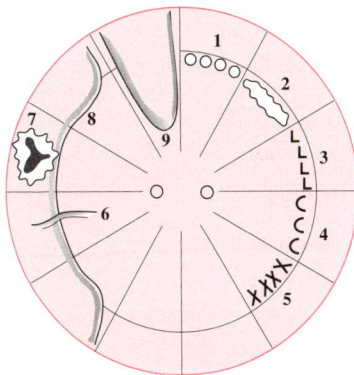

1. Xenon coagulation (one burn width apart)
2. Xenon coagulation (confluent burns)
3. Laser coagulation
4. Cryocoagulation
5. Diathermy coagulation

6. Radial retinal fold
7. Retinal break sealed with photocoagulation
8. Scleral buckling with circumferential seal
9. Scleral buckling with radial seal

DIABETIC RETINOPATHY: INTRODUCTION

RETINAL VASCULAR DISORDERS AND TUMOURS

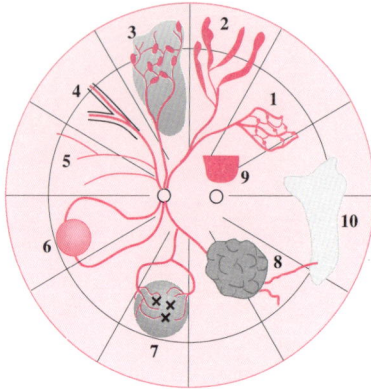

1. Vascular changes with micro-aneurysms
2. Intra- and pre-retinal neovascularization
3. Aneurysms and lipid deposits
4. Arterial attenuation
5. Obliterated vessels
6. Angiomatosis retinae
7. Retinoblastoma with calcification
8. Choroidal tumour
9. Preretinal haemorrhage
10. Vitreous haemorrhage

RISK FACTORS FOR DIABETIC RETINOPATHY

- After 30 years, 90% of diabetic patients will suffer from diabetic retinopathy (DR)
- Type I diabetic patients tend to develop proliferative DR (50% after 10–15 years), whereas type II diabetic patients tend to develop a maculopathy
- The risk of blindness is 10–20-fold higher in diabetic patients than in the general population
- After the occurrence of proliferations or epiretinal and vitreous haemorrhages, there is a 50% risk of blindness in the next five years
- Panretinal photocoagulation (PRP) prevents proliferative DR in 50% of cases
- Focal photocoagulation in focal maculopathy prevents visual deterioration in 50% of cases

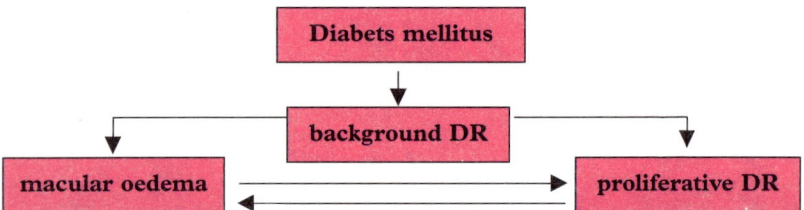

INFLUENTIAL FACTORS IN DIABETIC RETINOPATHY

Risk factors
Duration of diabetes
Patient's age
Short-term increase of insulin dosage
Pregnancy
Hypertension
Nephropathy
Hyperlipidaemia
Smoking
Cataract surgery (in advanced DR)
Rubeosis iridis

Protective factors
Chorioatrophic scars
High myopia
Optic atrophy
Good metabolic control

PATHOPHYSIOLOGY OF DIABETIC RETINAL CHANGES

Micro-aneurysms	Micro-outpouchings on the arteriolar and venular sides of the retinal capillary network; may leak fluid; many more micro-aneurysms are present microscopically and by fluorescein angiography than are seen clinically
Intraretinal microvascular abnormalities (IRMA)	Intraretinal arteriovenous shunts; no leakage on fluorescein angiogram; often adjacent to ischaemic zones
Neovascularization	Endothelial proliferation arising from the retinal veins. In contrast to IRMA, they cross other vessels and have a fibrous component. The optic nerve head is prone to neovascularizations, probably due to the absence of internal limiting membrane at this site
Haemorrhages	Blot and dot haemorrhages arise from microaneurysms and other capillary anomalies. They are located in the middle layers of the neuroretina
Nerve fibre layer haemorrhages	Follow the course of the retinal nerve fibres; flame-shaped appearance
Preretinal haemorrhages	Bleeding into the retrogel space (between the posterior face of the vitreous and the internal limiting membrane); often formation of an upper horizontal fluid level due to gravity; underlying vessels are obscured until absorption
Vitreous haemorrhages	Often spontaneous; slow absorption
Hard exudates	Yellowish deposits of lipid and lipoprotein due to abnormal vascular permeability, often formed in a circinate fashion
Cotton wool spots	Infarcts of nerve fibre layer due to capillary closure as a manifestation of microvascular ischaemia. Cotton wool spots result from an interruption of the axoplasmatic transport
Macular oedema	Results from increased capillary permeability; not always associated with reduced vision and often difficult to detect clinically in the early stages, but easily demonstrable with fundus fluorescein angiography

DIABETIC RETINOPATHY: CLASSIFICATION

NONPROLIFERATIVE RETINOPATHY

Mild	Microaneurysms
Moderate	• Intraretinal haemorrhages and/or
	• Microaneurysms and/or
	• Cotton wool spots
	• Irregular venous calibre
	• Intraretinal microvascular anomalies
High risk	Microaneurysms and intraretinal haemorrhages in all four quadrants
Advanced	In two or more quadrants:
	• Cotton wool spots
	• and irregular venous calibre
	• and intraretinal microvascular anomalies
High risk	Intraretinal microvascular anomalies in all four quadrants
	Marked irregular venous calibre in all four quadrants

PROLIFERATIVE RETINOPATHY

Early proliferative DR	Retinal neovascularizations not at disc but elsewhere (NVE)
High-risk proliferative DR	Epi- or peripapillary neovascularizations (NVD) with or without epiretinal haemorrhages or vitreous haemorrhages; or
	NVE with preretinal or vitreous haemorrhages

DEFINITION OF VISUAL LOSS AND RETINOPATHY ACCORDING TO ETDRS

[Results from the Early Treatment Diabetic Retinopathy Study (1991). *Ophthalmology* **98**:739–840]

Severe visual loss	Best corrected vision less than 3/60
Moderate visual loss	Visual loss of three Snellen lines
Mild/moderate retinopathy	Mild or moderate preproliferative DR
Severe retinopathy	Advanced preproliferative or early proliferative DR

DIABETIC RETINOPATHY: FOLLOW-UP

FOLLOW-UP IN PREPROLIFERATIVE RETINOPATHY

Fundus	Follow-up: type I diabetes mellitus	Follow-up: type II diabetes mellitus
No evidence of DR	annually; DR does not occur before puberty	As type I
Early preproliferative DR	6 months	12 months
Moderate preproliferative DR	3 months	6 months
Advanced preproliferative DR	2–3 months (PRP may be indicated)	As type I
Macular oedema without indication for treatment	3 months	As type I

RISK FACTORS FOR DIABETIC RETINOPATHY IN PREGNANCY

- Duration of diabetes mellitus before pregnancy
- Manifestation of hypertension
- Inadequate glucose monitoring (pregnancy in diabetes mellitus requires more frequent glucose monitoring)

PLANNED PREGNANCY IN DIABETES MELLITUS

- Inadequate blood glucose levels should be gradually normalized before pregnancy
- The presence of DR before pregnancy requires close monitoring; if needed, apply photocoagulation prior to or during the pregnancy

DIABETIC RETINOPATHY: MACULOPATHY

THE THREE TYPES OF DIABETIC MACULOPATHY AND THEIR FEATURES

Focal macular oedema (exudative maculopathy)	Zones of microaneurysms, intraretinal haemorrhages and hard exudates with oedema. The hard exudates often present in circular patterns around focal microvascular leakage.
Diffuse macular oedema (oedematous maculopathy)	Generalized macular oedema with diffuse capillary dilatation and relatively few focal changes.
Ischaemic maculopathy	Extensive capillary closure which is best demonstrated on fundus fluorescein angiography.

> Laser therapy for focal diabetic maculopathy should always be preceded by fluorescein angiography. The diagnosis of ischaemic maculopathy has to be confirmed with fluorescein angiography.

CLINICALLY SIGNIFICANT MACULAR OEDEMA

- thickening of the retina within 500 μm of the centre of the macula, and/or
- hard exudates within 500 μm of the centre of the macula, and/or
- zones of retinal thickening of one disc area (1500 μm) or larger, any part of which is within one disc diameter of the centre of the macula

DIABETIC RETINOPATHY: THERAPY

INDICATIONS FOR LASER THERAPY IN DR

	Indication	Treatment
Focal maculopathy	Focal macular changes within one disc diameter of the centre of the macula (not dependent on the visual acuity)	Direct photocoagulation of microaneurysms in the centre of circinate exudates and around haemorrhages; grid coagulation of oedematous zones
Diffuse maculopathy	Relative indication for laser coagulation (when clinically significant)	Grid treatment to the whole macula sparing the fovea and the papillomacular bundle
Severe pre-proliferative DR	Recommended	Panretinal photocoagulation, the worse eye first
Proliferative DR	Absolute indication	In the presence of a concomitant maculopathy, the macular changes should be treated first whereas the panretinal photocoagulation should be applied in a separate session

INDICATIONS FOR VITRECTOMY IN DR

• Severe, non-absorbing vitreous haemorrhage
• Traction retinal detachment
• Combined traction and rhegmatogenous retinal detachment
• Dense premacular haemorrhage (retrogel haemorrhage)
• Rubeosis iridis with vitreous opacity obscuring the view of the posterior pole
• Ghost-cell glaucoma
• Macular oedema with premacular traction
• Severe proliferative DR with a cataractous lens, which does not enable the application of laser therapy

POOR PROGNOSIS IN VITRECTOMY

• No adequate preceding laser therapy
• Optic nerve angiopathy
• Ischaemic macular oedema
• Surgical intervention carried out too late

DIABETIC RETINOPATHY: ARGON LASER PHOTOCOAGULATION

Panretinal coagulation	Dense	Diffuse
Spot size	500 μm	500 μm
Exposure time	0.1 sec	0.1 sec
Intensity	Moderate	Moderate
Number of burns	2000–3000	500–1200
Placement	$^1/_2$ burn-width apart; up to two disc diameters of the centre of the macula extending to the mid periphery and the equatorial retina	1 burn-width apart; up to two disc diameters of the centre of the macula extending to the mid periphery and the equatorial retina
Sessions	Two or more	One
Direct coagulation	NVE zones <2 disc diameters	NVE zones <2 disc diameters
Indication for subsequent treatment	NVE or high-risk proliferative DR (after 4 weeks)	NVE or high-risk proliferative DR (after 4 weeks)

Macular coagulation	Focal (direct)	Grid
Spot size	50–100 μm	<200 μm
Exposure time	0.05–0.1 sec	0.05–0.1 sec
Intensity	Whitening or darkening of the microaneurysms to be obtained (80–120 mW)	Mild (80–180 mW)
Number of burns	Sufficient to coagulate all leaking foci	All zones of diffuse leakage
Placement	500–3000 μm from the centre of the macula	500–3000 μm from the centre of the macula, sparing the papillomacular bundle
Sessions	One	One ·
Indication for subsequent treatment	Clinical significant macular oedema and further lesions that require treatment (after ≥3 months)	Clinical significant macular oedema and further lesions that require treatment (after ≥3 months)

[Results from the Early Treatment Diabetic Retinopathy Study (1991). *Ophthalmology* **98**:739–840]

The above data apply for the use of argon green (514 nm) and a Goldmann 3 mirror lens in clear media. When using a panfundoscopic lens, the spot size is reduced from 500 to 300 μm because of the approximately 1.5-fold magnification compared with the Goldmann levels.

Argon green (514 nm) should be chosen over argon blue–green (488 nm), because the shorter wavelength is better absorbed by the macular xanthophyll and may therefore cause foveal damage.

CENTRAL RETINAL VEIN OCCLUSION (CRVO)

DIFFERENTIAL DIAGNOSIS OF (CRVO)

Recent CRVO
Anterior ischaemic optic neuropathy

Papilloedema

Hypertensive retinopathy

Diabetic retinopathy

Hyperviscosity syndrome

Old CRVO
Dry macular degeneration

NVD

FEATURES OF ISCHAEMIC CRVO

Fundus	•	$\geq$10 cotton wool spots; dark, blotchy retinal
	•	haemorrhages
Slit lamp	+	Rubeosis iridis
Vision	−	<6/60
Swinging flashlight test	•	Relative afferent pupillary defect
Fluorescein angiography	•	Areas of capillary nonperfusion (>1 disc diameter), maximum venous filling $\geq$20 sec
Visual field	−	Constricting defects, relative central scotoma
ERG	−	b-wave $\downarrow$, b/a-amplitude $\downarrow$, retinal sensitivity $\downarrow$

+ diagnosis confirmed; • significant feature; − less significant feature

CRVO WITH POOR PROGNOSIS

• Ischaemic
• Cystoid macular oedema
• Dense, dark, blotchy haemorrhages
• Visual acuity <6/60
• Uncontrolled hypertension
• Diabetes mellitus
• Old age

INDICATIONS FOR PANRETINAL PHOTOCOAGULATION IN CRVO

CRVO is considered ischaemic if:
• FFA demonstrates retinal nonperfusion or in the presence of two or more of the following:

- More than 10 cotton wool spots
- Extensive haemorrhages
- Maximum venous filling (t_{mvf}) $\geqslant 20$ sec
- Visual acuity <6/60

Indication for PRP:
- Ischaemic CRVO
- Rubeosis iridis

Application:
- 2000–3000 500 μm burns

CENTRAL RETINAL ARTERY OCCLUSION (CRAO)

CAUSES OF CENTRAL ARTERY OCCLUSION

Emboli
Hypertension (arteriosclerotic plaques)
Carotid artery stenosis
Mitral valve disease
Endocarditis
Mural thrombi following myocardial infarction
Lipid emboli (Purtscher's retinopathy, pancreatitis)
Calcific emboli

Vaso-obliteration
Giant cell arteritis
Connective-tissue diseases
Clotting disorders
Optic nerve drüsen
Sickle cell anaemia
Homocystinuria
Contraceptives

Compression
Raised intraocular pressure (acute angle-closure glaucoma, retrobulbar haematoma)

MANAGEMENT OF CENTRAL RETINAL ARTERY OCCLUSION

Diagnosis
Vision, visual field, fundoscopy, erythrocyte sedimentation rate, full blood count, haematocrit, blood clotting, fasting glucose, blood pressure, carotid Doppler ultrasound and medical opinion

Therapy
Ocular massage and intravenous acetazolamide to lower the intra-ocular pressure, anterior chamber paracentesis, 95% oxygen

OCULAR MASSAGE IN CENTRAL ARTERY VEIN OCCLUSION

- Patient should lie flat to avoid orthostatic reduced retinal perfusion
- Digital massage is applied through the closed upper lid
- The massage should be applied intermittently, gently increasing each time, and discontinued promptly after 3–5 seconds
- Depending on the patient's compliance, ocular massage may be self-applied

HYPERTENSIVE RETINOPATHY

GRADING OF FUNDUS CHANGES IN HYPERTENSION

[Keith NM, Wagener HP, Barker NW (1939) Some different types of essential hypertension. Their course and prognosis. *Am J Med Sci* **197**:332–343]

	Optic nerve head	Retinal arteries	Retina
Grade I	No abnormal finding	Arterial attenuation with abnormal light reflex from the arterial wall	No abnormal finding
Grade II	No abnormal finding	As above but also irregular arterial calibre and venous nipping (Salus' sign)	Haemorrhages, hard exudates with possible macular star formation
Grade III	Early disc swelling (begins nasally)	As above but also advanced arterial constriction	As above but also cotton wool spots
Grade IV	Established swelling of the optic nerve head	As in stage III	Oedema

FUNDUS CHANGES IN MALIGNANT HYPERTENSION

[Hayreh SS (1989) Classification of hypertensive fundus changes and their order of appearance. *Ophthalmologica* **198**:247–260]

- Hypertensive retinopathy
- Hypertensive choroidopathy
- Hypertensive optic neuropathy

UPPER LIMITS OF THE BLOOD PRESSURE IN ADULTS

	Systolic	Diastolic
Up to 64 years old	140 mmHg	90 mmHg
Over 64 years old	160 mmHg	90 mmHg

Mild hypertension	Diastolic BP 90–104 mmHg
Moderate hypertension	Diastolic BP 105–114 mmHg
Severe hypertension	Diastolic BP >114 mmHg

RETINAL DETACHMENT

PROGRESSION OF SUBRETINAL FLUID (SRF) ACCUMULATION

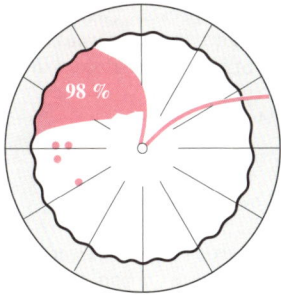

SRF spreading temporarily or superonasally: 98% of primary retinal breaks are located within an area of $1^1/_2$ clock hours from the upper border of the retinal detachment

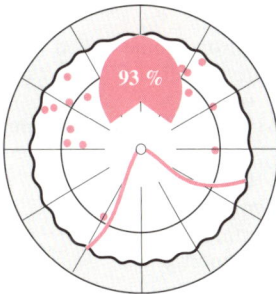

SRF spreading in the upper circumference: 93% of primary retinal breaks are located in a triangle, one tip of which is situated at 12 o'clock and the others $1^1/_2$ clock hours right and left from the vertical meridian, reaching the equator

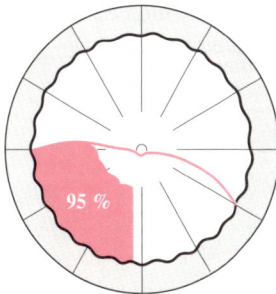

SRF spreading in the lower quadrants: 95% of primary retinal breaks are located between 6 o'clock and the highest border of the retinal detachment

RETINOSCHISIS

RETINOSCHISIS VERSUS RETINAL DETACHMENT

	Retinoschisis	Rhegmatogenous retinal detachment
Transparency	Transparent	Reduced transparency
Mobility	None	Wavy movements on moving the globe (fundoscopy, ultrasound)
Hyperpigmentation	Uncommon	Demarcation line (after weeks to months)
Retinal breaks	May occur in the inner or outer layers of the schisis (nonprogressive in most cases)	Always present (without treatment, accumulation of subretinal fluid will progress)
Site of formation	More common inferotemporally than superotemporally	More common superotemporally than inferotemporally
Manifestation	Usually bilateral	Usually monocular
Refraction	Often hypermetropia	Often myopia
Visual field	Absolute scotoma	Relative scotoma, later absolute scotoma

ACQUIRED RETINOSCHISIS VERSUS CONGENITAL RETINOSCHISIS

	Acquired	Congenital
Aetiology	Degenerative	X-chromosome linked
Age of onset	Usually over 50 years of age	Early childhood (2–5 years of age)
Symptoms	Usually asymptomatic and nonprogressive	Mild deterioration of vision, strabismus, vitreous haemorrhage
Maculopathy	Rarely	Typical 'cartwheel' maculopathy
Vitreous haemorrhage	Rarely	Common
Manifestation	Usually bilateral	Always bilateral
Progression	The reticular, less common type, may progress to the posterior pole	Slowly progressive deterioration during childhood, stationary thereafter

PROLIFERATIVE VITREORETINOPATHY (PVR)

CLASSIFICATION OF PROLIFERATIVE VITREORETINOPATHY (PVR)

[The Retina Society Terminology Committee (1983) The classification of retinal detachment with proliferative vitreoretinopathy. *Ophthalmology* **90**:121–125]

Grade	Degree	Signs and symptoms
A	Slight	Vitreous opacity, pigment clumps in the vitreous humour, vascular proliferation on the posterior vitreous surface
B	Mild	Wrinkling of the posterior vitreous surface, PVR membranes, rolled edges of retinal breaks, vascular tortuosity
C	Moderate	Tractional retinal detachment
• C1		• in one quadrant
• C2		• in two quadrants
• C3		• in three quadrants
D	Severe	Circumferential retinal detachment
• D1		• with wide cone-shaped opening
• D2		• with narrow cone-shaped opening
• D3		• without view of the disc (closed cone)

STAGING OF PVR-ACCORDING TO MACHEMER *ET AL.*

[Machemer R *et al.* (1991) An updated classification of retinal detachment with proliferative vitreoretinopathy. *Am J Ophthamol* **112**:159–165]

Grade	Signs and symptoms
A	Vitreous haemorrhage, pigment clumps in the vitreous humour and on the inner retinal surface
B	Inner retinal surface folds; immobile retina; rolled and irregular edges of retinal breaks; vascular tortuosity; reduced vitreous mobility
C P 1–12	Posterior to the equator: retinal fold formation★; subretinal strands★
C A 1–12	Anterior to the equator: retinal fold formation★; subretinal strands★; opaque vitreous humour with formation of strands

★Location to be noted using clock hours

TYPE OF CONTRACTIONS IN PVR GRADE C

Type	Location	Characteristics
Focal	Posterior	Star folds posterior to the vitreous humour
Diffuse	Posterior	Confluent star folds posterior to the vitreous humour; disc occasionally covered
Subretinal	Posterior/ anterior	Subretinal proliferations; circular strand formation near the disc; 'moth eaten'-like defects
Circumferential	Anterior	Contraction along the posterior border of the vitreous base; stretching of the peripheral retina; posterior, radial retinal fold formation
Anterior displacement	Anterior	Anterior displacement of the vitreous base by proliferative tissue; ciliary body processes visible; iris deformation

VITRECTOMY

Within 1 week	Endophthalmitis Acute chalcosis Severe trauma (reconstruction of the globe with injection of silicone oil)
After 1–2 weeks	Secondary vitrectomy after primary reconstruction following trauma
Later than 3 weeks	Severe persistent vitreous haemorrhage

CAUSES OF EPIRETINAL GLIOSIS ('MACULAR PUCKER')

- Idiopathic
- Retinal detachment surgery
- Photocoagulation
- Untreated retinal defects
- Retinal vascular disease (DR, vein occlusion, Eales' disease)
- Intraocular inflammation (uveitis, perforating eye injury)
- Retinitis pigmentosa

VITREORETINAL DEGENERATIONS

CLASSIFICATION OF PERIPHERAL RETINAL DEGENERATIONS

Primary trophic changes	Senile (acquired) retinoschisis Paving stone degeneration Snailtrack and lattice degeneration Equatorial degeneration Degenerative round holes
Developmental changes	'White without pressure' Retinal tufts (tags), meridional folds
Tractional changes	Rosette-shaped tractions Reactive pigment epithelium proliferation Operculate retinal tears U-shaped retinal tears

BENIGN VARIATIONS IN THE ORA SERRATA

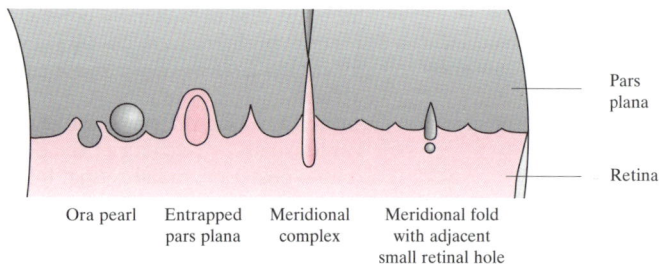

Ora pearl — Entrapped pars plana — Meridional complex — Meridional fold with adjacent small retinal hole — Pars plana — Retina

BENIGN PERIPHERAL RETINAL DEGENERATIONS AND PREDISPOSING CHANGES

Predisposing changes
Lattice degeneration

Snailtrack

Zonular traction retinal tufts

Benign changes
Microcystic degeneration

'White without pressure'

Chorioretinal degeneration (paving stone)

Ectopic ciliary epithelium

Noncystic retinal tufts

Cystic retinal tufts

Meridional complexes

Snowflakes

RISK FACTORS (IN ORDER OF SIGNIFICANCE) OF TRACTIONAL RETINAL DETACHMENT DUE TO VITREORETINAL DEGENERATIONS

- Atrophic round holes
- Retinal tear with traction
- Tractional retinal detachment in the other eye
- High myopia
- Aphakia

INDICATIONS FOR PROPHYLACTIC TREATMENT

Lesion	Prophylatic treatment is indicated in
Lattice degeneration without atrophic hole formation	Aphakia Pseudophakia History of retinal detachment in the other eye
Lattice degeneration with atrophic hole formation	Aphakia Pseudophakia History of retinal detachment in the other eye Myopia (>3 dpt) Symptomatic posterior vitreous detachment
Operculate retinal tears • with vitreoretinal traction • without vitreoretinal traction	• All cases • Aphakia, pseudophakia, location in the upper circumference, symptomatic posterior vitreous detachment, vitreous haemorrhage, myopia (>3 dpt)
Zonular traction retinal tufts	Aphakia
Snailtrack with large atrophic round holes	All cases
U-shaped tears	All cases
Atraumatic giant tears	Circumferential prophylactic treatment of the other eye

RETINITIS PIGMENTOSA

CLINICAL FEATURES OF RETINAL PIGMENTOSA (RP)

Fundus

Arteriolar attenuation	Almost always
Waxy optic disc	Almost always
Macular changes	Almost always
Abnormal macular reflex	Almost always
Cystoid macular oedema	20–30% of advanced cases
RPE changes, initial depigmentation, bone-spicule pigmentation (3–5 years after commencement of symptoms)	Almost always

Anterior segment

Vitreous condensation	~100%
Myopia	Frequent
Cataract (over 40 years of age; subcapsular, posterior)	Common

Inheritance

Autosomal dominant	~25% (best prognosis)
Sporadic	~47% (next best prognosis)
Autosomal recessive	~20% (association with systemic disorders)
X-linked recessive	~8% (worst prognosis)

Diffuse, type 1 autosomal dominant RP versus regional, type 2 autosomal dominant RP

Type 1 (D-type)	Diffuse early loss of the rod sensitivity
	Delayed onset of cone dysfunction
	Progressive constricting scotomata
Type 2 (R-type)	Regional rod and cone dysfunction
	Delayed onset of nyctalopia
	Slow-progressive peripheral visual field defect

The use of ERG to exclude RP

RP may be considered excluded, if ERG is normal in:
- recessive cases after 6 years of age
- dominant cases after 16 years of age

1. Medical history

- Hearing loss (e.g. Usher's syndrome)
- Neurological defects (ataxia, epilepsy, mental retardation)
- Infection (tuberculosis, Rubella)
- Medication (nonsteroidal anti-inflammatory drugs, chloroquine, antidepressant drugs, anti-epilectics)

2. Ophthalmic history

First glasses (myopia), nyctalopia, visual field defects (difficulty in walking downstairs), colour vision

3. Family history

History of RP

4. Baseline ophthalmic examination

Lid malformations, mortility, pupillary responses, visual acuity, refraction, intra-ocular pressure

5. Biomicroscopy

Corneal abnormalities, lens opacity,
Vitreous cell or fibrillar changes, posterior
vitreous detachment (PVD)

6. Fundoscopy

Waxy optic disc, arteriolar attenuation, bone-spicule pigmentation in the retinal mid periphery, tapetal reflex, macular oedema

7. Perimetry

Visual field defects

8. Colour vision

Colour vision defects

9. Dark adaptation

Available only in large centres; provides valuable information especially in atypical RP

10. Electrophysiology

Scotopic ERG (changes already demonstrable in the early stages of the disease)

11. Genetic counselling

Genetic counselling must be given prior to planning a family

RETINOPATHY OF PREMATURITY

TERMINOLOGY

Full-term	Birth between 38 and 42 gestational weeks
Premature	Birth before the end of the 37th week of gestation (260 days)
Prematurity signs	Length <48 cm
	Body weight <2500 g
ROP high risk	Body weight <1250 g (of premature infants weighing less than 750 g at birth, 90% develop some degree of ROP)

[Cryotherapy for Retinopathy of Prematurity Group (1991). *Arch Ophthalmol* **98**:1628–1640]

INTERNATIONAL CLASSIFICATION OF RETINOPATHY OF PREMATURITY (ROP)

[Committee for the Classification of Retinopathy of Prematurity (1987). *Arch Opthalmol* **105**:906–913]

Stage	Changes
1	Demarcation line
2	Ridge
3	Ridge with extraretinal fibrovascular proliferation
4	Subtotal retinal detachment
	4a extrafoveal
	4b retinal detachment including fovea
5	Total retinal detachment
'Plus' disease	Dilatation and tortuosity of the peripheral retinal vessels

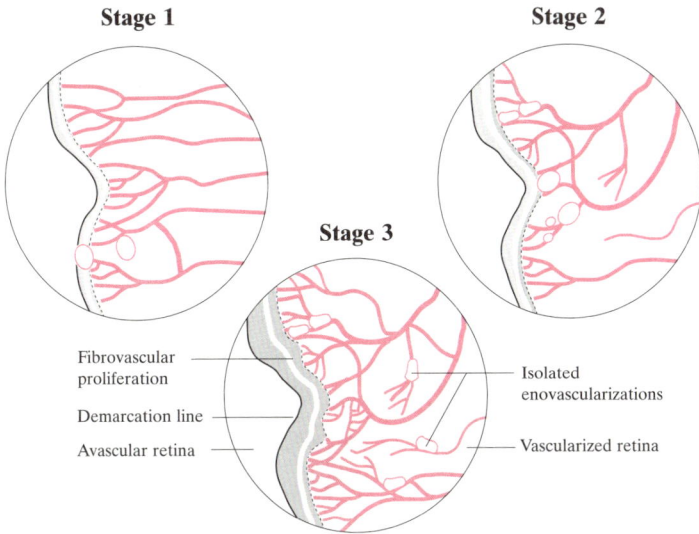

Stage 1

Stage 2

Stage 3

Fibrovascular proliferation

Demarcation line

Avascular retina

Isolated enovascularizations

Vascularized retina

INDICATIONS FOR OPHTHALMIC EXAMINATION

Premature infants	Birth weight below 1500 g
	Essential even if over 1500 g but O_2 therapy with >30% O_2
Premature and full-term infants	O_2 therapy with >30% O_2 for >2 days
	PaO_2 >100 mmHg
Initial examination	32–34th gestational week (4–5 weeks old)
Last examination (in previously undetected abnormalities)	Between birth and 10 weeks old

The earlier the manifestation of ROP changes, the worse the prognosis

TREATMENT

Stage 1   Fundoscopy every 2 weeks
Stage 2   Fundoscopy once weekly
Stage 3   Cryotherapy or laser photocoagulation
Stage 4   Scleral buckling, vitrectomy (but treatment is not usually
           recommended because of poor prognosis)

RETINAL ZONES

Zone I   Posterior area centred on the disc, which extends twice the
             distance from the disc to the centre of the macula in all
             directions
Zone II   Includes the area centred on the disc, with a radius equal to the
             distance to the nasal ora serrata
Zone III   Temporal periphery (most common location for early ROP
             changes)

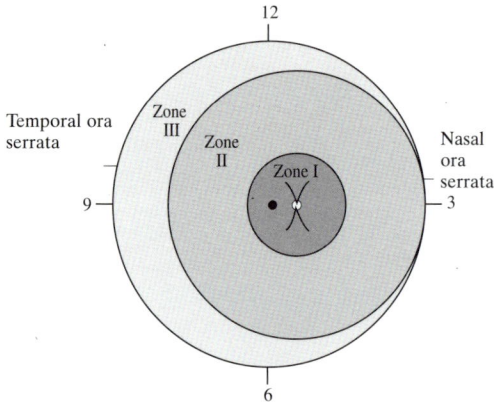

DIFFERENTIAL DIAGNOSIS OF RETINOBLASTOMA

	Retinoblastoma	PHPV*	ROP	Coats' disease
Bilaterality	$^2/_3$ unilateral $^1/_3$ bilateral	Usually unilateral	Almost always bilateral	Practically always unilateral
Globe size	–	Microphthalmus	–	–
Age at manifestation	18 months	Neonatal period	Premature infants	1st decade
History	6% of cases have positive family history	–	Prematurity, O_2 therapy	–
Clinical features	Leukocoria, calcification (best detectable with ultrasound or CT)	Elongated ciliary processes, no calcifications	Proliferative retinopathy	(Most commonly boys (3:1 = M:F); exudates, vascular dilatation and tortuosity

*Persistent hyperplastic primary vitreous

INHERITANCE

- Approximately 95% of all retinoblastoma cases are sporadic. All bilateral sporadic retinoblastoma patients are considered to have germinal mutation and are therefore gene carriers; 15% of unilateral sporadic retinoblastoma cases are also the result of germinal mutation.
- Nonsporadic retinoblastoma is due to autosomal dominant inheritance with 90% penetrance (10% of carriers remain unaffected).
- Hereditary retinoblastoma is a risk factor for developing other cancers later in life, the most common of which is osteosarcoma. Bilateral retinoblastoma and pinealoblastoma is called 'trilateral retinoblastoma'.
- The presence of retinoblastoma in childhood and osteosarcoma later in life strongly suggests a germinal mutation.
- If two or more family members are affected (multiplex disease), DNA studies to disclose the retinoblastoma gene with the germinal mutation are indicated. Other family members who share the presumably mutant copy of the retinoblastoma gene are also at risk for the disease.
- A proved mutation indicates examination under general anaesthesia of the carrier's offspring. On the other hand, negative DNA studies obviate the need for general anaesthesia in a young child.

GENETIC COUNSELLING IN RETINOBLASTOMA: THE RISK FOR SUBSEQUENT CHILDREN

Familial cases

- If the index patient and one or more family members are affected, the risk for each of the index patient's children developing retinoblastoma is 45%
- If the index patient is asymptomatic with one of his/her parents a known carrier, the risk for the index patient's children developing retinoblastoma is 4.5%
- If one child has already developed retinoblastoma, the risk for the other siblings becoming affected is 45%

Sporadic cases

- If retinoblastoma affects only the index patient: in unilateral cases (no germinal mutation), the risk for the index patient's children developing retinoblastoma is 6.5%; in bilateral cases, the risk for the children developing the disease is 45%
- If the index patient is asymptomatic, but one of the children already has bilateral retinoblastoma, the risk for the other siblings becoming affected is 2.5%
- If the index patient is asymptomatic, but one of the children already has unilateral retinoblastoma, the risk for the other siblings becoming affected is <1%

MACULAR DISEASE

LEVEL OF DYSFUNCTION

Nerve fibre layer   Juvenile retinoschisis (X-chromosome linked)

Photoreceptors   Autosomal dominant cone dystrophy
Stargardt's disease

Pigment epithelium   Central serous retinopathy
Best's disease (vitelliform macular dystrophy)
Central areolar choroidal dystrophy
Progressive foveal dystrophy
Benign concentric annular macular dystrophy
Stargardt's disease (fundus flavimaculatus)
Sjögren's dystrophy of the retinal pigment epithelium
(RPE)

Bruch's membrane   Age-related macular degeneration
Myopic maculopathy
Angioid streaks
Familial drüsen (Doyne's honeycomb dystrophy)

Choroid   Choroidal folds
Central areolar choroidal dystrophy
Sorsby's pseudo-inflammatory macular dystrophy
North Carolina macular dystrophy

CHLOROQUINE MACULOPATHY

Ophthalmic side-effects of chloroquine   Abnormal accommodation
Reversible corneal opacity
Irreversible retinal changes

Symptoms of chloroquine maculopathy   Reduction of visual acuity
Abnormal dark adaptation
Colour vision defects
Visual field defects
Concentric hyper- and hypopigmentation
macular changes (bull's eye maculopathy)

Fluorescence angiography   Window defect corresponds to the
hypopigmentation

Expected manifestation of chloroquine maculopathy   When the daily dosage of chloroquine
exceeds 250 mg daily

Electrophysiology   EOG: reduced light peak
ERG: increased A-wave, reduced B-wave

SYNOPSIS OF DOMINANT MACULAR DYSTROPHIES

Disease	Ophthalmoscopy	Visual acuity	Electrophysiology
Best's disease (vitelliform macular dystrophy)	Disease of pigment epithelium; 'Egg-yolk' maculopathy during the second decade of life, later pseudohypopyon and 'scrambled egg' appearance	Visual impairment in the late stages of the disease	EOG abnormal during all stages
Autosomal dominant cone dystrophy	'Bull's-eye' maculopathy, later RP-like changes	Poor visual acuity starting early in the second decade of life; photophobia	ERG abnormal
Progressive foveal dystrophy	Disease of pigment epithelium	Marked visual impairment often in the first decade of life	Normal cone and rod ERG and normal EOG
Familial hyaline deposits (Doyne's honeycomb dystrophy, malattia léventinese)	Disseminated hyaline deposits on Bruch's membrane	Visual impairment in middle age	Normal ERG and EOG
Central areolar pigment epithelial dystrophy*	RPE atrophy	Mild visual impairment	Normal ERG and EOG
Central areolar choroidal dystrophy*	Choroidal atrophy with secondary atroph of the pigment epithelium	Slow-progressive visual loss	Normal ERG and EOG in early stages
Sorsby's pseudo-inflammatory macular dystrophy	Disease of pigment epithelium, choroidal neovascular membranes, subretinal haemorrhages	Loss of central vision with progressive impairment of peripheral vision	Normal ERG and EOG

Disease	Ophthalmoscopy	Visual acuity	Electrophysiology
Butterfly-shaped RPE dystrophy	Symmetrical macular hyperpigmentation	Slight, non-progressive visual impairment	Normal ERG, subnormal EOG
Benign concentric annular macular dystrophy	'Bull's-eye' maculopathy	Slight, non-progressive visual impairment	ERG and EOG usually normal
Dominant Stargardt's disease	Bronze, irregular shaped macular lesions at the level of the RPE	Deterioration of vision in the second decade of life, initially without visible fundal changes	ERG and EOG normal in early stages

*Probably variations of the same disease

ACQUIRED MACULAR DISEASE

SUBRETINAL NEOVASCULARIZATIONS (SRN) MAY OCCUR IN:

- Exudative age-related macular degeneration
- Myopic maculopathy
- Chorioretinal scars
- Rubella retinopathy
- Best's disease (vitelliform macular dystrophy)
- Serpiginous choroidopathy
- Acute posterior multifocal placoid pigment epitheliopathy (APMPPE)
- Papillary drüsen
- Choroidal rupture
- Angioid streaks
- RPE hamartoma
- Presumed ocular histoplasmosis
- Idiopathic posterior SRN
- After photocoagulation

STAGES OF IDIOPATHIC MACULAR HOLE FORMATION

[Gass JDM (1988) Idiopathic senile macular hole: its early stages and pathogenesis. *Arch Ophthalmol* **106**:629–639]

Stage	Features	Visual acuity
I ('impending hole')		
A	Foveal yellow spot; decreased or absent foveal depression; no Watzke's sign*, foveal detachment (100–200 μm)	Visual impairment between $^6/_9$ and $^6/_{24}$

Stage	Features	Visual acuity
B	Foveal yellow ring; decreased or absent foveal depression; no Watzke's sign★, foveal detachment ($>200\,\mu m$)	
II (early macular hole)	Eccentric early full-thickness macular hole	Between $^6/_{12}$ and $^6/_{36}$
III (fully developed macular hole)	Full-thickness macular hole with yellow deposits at the level of the RPE within the hole; pseudo-operculum (condensation of vitreous humour); positive Watzke's sign★; diameter $\sim500\,\mu m$	Between $^6/_{36}$ and $^3/_{60}$
IV (macular hole with posterior vitreous detachment)	As stage III, but with posterior vitreous detachment	

★ Watzke's sign refers to an interruption of the slit beam focused on the hole

CAUSES OF CYSTOID MACULAR OEDEMA

- Diabetic retinopathy
- Retinal vein occlusion
- Uveitis
- Hypertensive retinopathy
- Retinal telangiectasias (Coats' disease, juxtafoveolar telangiectasia)
- Macroaneurysm
- Hereditary retinal dystrophies
- Epiretinal gliosis
- Intraocular tumours (malignant melanoma, choroidal haemangioma)
- Choroidal neovascularizations age-related macular degeneration, angioid streaks)
- After intraocular surgery (Irvine–Gass syndrome)

RETINOPATHY IN BLOOD DISORDERS

BLOOD DISORDERS WHICH MAY BE ASSOCIATED WITH RETINAL CHANGES

- **Anaemia** (retinal changes more likely to occur with a haemoglobin of $<6.5\,g/dl$ and thrombocytopenia)
- **Leukaemia**
- **Polycythaemia vera** and **secondary polycythaemia** (retinopathy more likely in primary polycythaemia)
- **Dysproteinaemia** (e.g. Waldenström's macroglobulinaemia)
- **Sickle-cell retinopathy**

Note:
1. Retinal changes in the above blood disorders may include retinal haemorrhages, white-centred retinal haemorrhages (Roth's spots), cotton wool spots, retinal oedema, venous dilatation and tortuosity.
2. Retinal changes in polycythaemia often include optic disc hyperaemia.
3. Mid periphery salmon-patch haemorrhages and the disc sign of sickling (red spots and lines on disc) are typical of sickle-cell retinopathy. Proliferative retinopathy may occur as the most severe complication of sickle-cell disease.

RETINAL CAPILLARY HAEMANGIOMA

History
Retinal capillary haemangioma may be associated with systemic lesions. It is then referred to as **von Hippel–Lindau syndrome**. When seen by an ophthalmologist, it is therefore important to arrange for neurological referral to exclude systemic tumours. Due to the autosomal dominant inheritance, screening of the relatives should also be undertaken. Medical opinion, in particular with reference to renal and suprarenal involvement, should also be obtained.

Investigations
- Blood pressure
- Abdominal ultrasound (kidneys, adrenal bodies, pancreas)
- 24-hour urine (vanillylmandelic acid level)
- Ophthalmoscopy with mydriasis
- Fluorescein angiography
- CT imaging of the brain
- CT imaging of the abdomen

Secondary changes in retinal capillary haemangioma
- Subretinal exudation, exudative retinal detachment
- Vitreous haemorrhage
- Subretinal neovascularization
- Proliferative vitreoretinopathy and formation of epiretinal membrane
- Traction retinal detachment

Classification
I	Angioma up to $^1/_2$ disc diameter
II	Angioma $^1/_2$–2 disc diameters
IIa	without secondary changes
IIb	with secondary changes
III	Angioma >2 disc diameters
IIIa	without secondary changes
IIIb	with secondary changes
IV	Angioma on disc or juxtapapillary

Chapter 10

OPTIC NERVE/VISUAL PATHWAYS

GENERAL CONSIDERATIONS IN THE CLINICAL EVALUATION OF THE OPTIC NERVE HEAD

VALUABLE DIFFERENTIAL DIAGNOSTIC SIGNS

Finding	Interpretation
Spontaneous venous pulsation	Present in 80% of normal subjects; ceases if intracranial pressure >200 mmHg
Extent of optic disc excavation (cup)	Glaucoma follow-up
Asymmetrical optic discs	Glaucoma in Foster–Kennedy syndrome
Disc pallor	Pale disc in optic atrophy
Hyperaemia	Early papilloedema
Blurred disc margin	Early sign for swelling of the nerve fibres
Peripapillary capillary dilatation without leakage on the fluorescein angiography	Typically seen in Leber's hereditary optic neuropathy
Flame-shaped haemorrhages	Haemorrhages in the nerve fibre layer; seen in swelling of the optic nerve head, but also in glaucoma
Cells in the posterior vitreous	Juxtapapillary chorioretinitis
Peripapillarly choroidal atrophy	Malperfusion of the peripapillary retina
Ridged optic nerve head with very small or absent excavation and abnormal vascular architecture	Optic nerve drusen
Paton's lines	Retinal folds on the temporal side of the disc due to swelling of the optic nerve head
Unilateral swelling of the optic nerve head with visual loss	Typical presentation of papillitis, anterior ischaemic optic neuropathy, juxtapapillary chorioretinitis
Optic atrophy with temporal hemianopic defects	Typical in chiasmal lesions (usually compressing)

PAPILLOEDEMA/SWOLLEN OPTIC NERVE HEAD

DIFFERENTIAL DIAGNOSIS

Papilloedema	Due to raised intracranial pressure (e.g. congenital aqueduct stenosis, posterior fossa tumours, pseudotumour cerebri); bilateral, although often asymmetrical; no acute visual loss; total length cylindrical-type thickening of optic nerve on CT/MRI
Papilloedema with preretinal haemorrhages	If located in front of the macula, it gives rise to severe decrease of vision; in adults almost always indicative of a subarachnoid haemorrhage (Terson's syndrome), in infants of subdural haemorrhage
Pseudopapilloedema due to optic disc drusen	Abnormal vascular architecture; enlargement of the blind spot; may cause field defects, sometimes haemorrhages calcification is seen on ultrasound; Optic disc drusden are hyaline deposits in the optic nerve head, typically demonstrable on pre-injection photographs autofluorescence (L)
Pseudopapilloedema of hypermetropia	Usually in children with moderate to high hypermetropia; no enlargement of blind spot
Epipapillary membrane (Bergmeister's papilla)	If the atrophy of the hyaloid artery is incomplete and the epipapillary membrane in front of the disc is dense enough, it may be misinterpreted as disc oedema
Central retinal vein occlusion (CRVO)	Typically presents with retinal vein tortuosity, disc swelling and haemorrhages even in the peripheral fundus; cotton wool spots are uncommon in nonischaemic CRVO, but usually present in ischaemic CRVO
Papillophlebitis	Unilateral in young healthy adults; mild visual impairment; disc swelling; moderate amount of retinal haemorrhages; good prognosis; consider optic disc vasculitis or CRVO in young adults
Malignant hypertensive retinopathy	Attenuated arteries and disc swelling followed by haemorrhages and infarction
Hypotony	Postoperatively or following trauma; IOP in the range of 2–4 mmHg; mild swelling of disc and macula
Optic nerve glioma	Usually in young children; 55% of cases are associated with neurofibromatosis; CT/MRI shows encapsulated mass with identical densities of nerve and tumour
Optic nerve meningioma	Typically middle-aged women; CT/MRI shows irregular margins of mass and excludes glioma (negative optic nerve in contrast to the density of the tumour)

Infiltrative optic neuropathy	Consider haematological disorders as lymphoma or leukaemia, but also granulomatous infiltrative diseases (e.g. sarcoid, tuberculosis)
Juxtapapillary choroiditis	Focal chorioretinitis next and usually temporal to the disc; the rest of the disc remains normal; cells in the vitreous; unlikely to be confused with papilloedema which always begins on the nasal margin of the disc
Leber's stellate neuroretinitis	Disc swelling and macular star due to juxtapapillary retinal detachment; query aetiology; often bilateral
Leber's optic atrophy	Rare; hereditary; 85% are young men; peripapillary capillary dilatation without leakage on fluorescein angiography; frequently begins as unilateral papillitis but becomes bilateral soon after; disc atrophy follows a few weeks later; diagnosis by molecular genetics
Optic Neuritis	Afferent pupillary defect; visual loss, defective colour vision and central field defects. CT indicated, MRI may show enhancement and barrier defects of involved section of optic nerve; ocular movements not restricted, but produce slight to moderate pain; CT appearance as papilloedema, but normal optic nerve head
Uveitis	May cause disc swelling, especially intermediate uveitis
Drug-induced optic neuropathy	Sudden vision loss; disc normal or swollen typically caused by methanol isoniazid or streptomycin; prognosis is good once the drug is stopped
Toxic amblyopia	Poor nutrition, often in combination with excessive amounts of tobacco and alcohol; gradual, bilateral deterioration of vision; centrocaecal scotomata; disc oedema good prognosis in early cases
Big blind-spot syndrome	Mild swelling of the optic nerve head may be present; visual acuity remains unaffected
Arteritic anterior ischaemic optic neuropathy (AION)	A manifestation of giant cell arteritis; patient usually over 70 years of age; visual loss is sudden and in some cases bilateral; the visual loss is frequently accompanied by periocular pain and preceding headaches, jaw claudication and polymyalgia rheumatica; raised erythrocyte sedimentation rate; raised C-reactive protein. A temporal artery biopsy is often done to confine diarposis in view of the need for long-term steroids
Nonarteritic AION	Patient is 45–65 years of age (about 10 years younger than arteritic AION), otherwise healthy or with a history of systemic vascular disease such as hypertension; loss of vision is sudden, rarely bilateral and some may have diffuse periocular pain, but otherwise painless, the fellow eye commonly has a

small or absent optic cup; prognosis for visual rehabilitation is better than in arteritic AION; one-third of patients develop AION in the seond eye within two years

THE STAGES OF PAPILLOEDEMA

Early papilloedema

- Hyperaemia
- Slight obliteration of the disc cup (difficult to confirm unless the patient's cup/disc ratio was previously determined)
- Blurring of the nasal disc margin
- Blurring of the peripapillary nerve fibre layer
- Absent spontaneous venous pulsation*
- Visual acuity remains unchanged
- Blind spot may be enlarged

Chronic papilloedema

- Regression of the hyperaemia and haemorrhages
- Lipid deposits under the nerve fibre layer
- Visual acuity often affected in the eye with the more marked disc swelling
- Paton's lines

Established papilloedema

- Increased hyperaemia
- Increased filling in of the optic cup
- Prominent optic nerve head
- Blurring of all the disc margins
- Peripapillary haemorrhages
- Venostasis
- Cotton wool spots
- Retinal folds on the temporal side of the disc (the folds disappear later due to increased oedema)
- Transient visual obscuration (TVO)
- Enlarged blind spot

Atrophic papilloedema

- Disc pallor
- Blurred disc margin
- Regressed disc swelling
- Reduced visual acuity

*The presence of spontaneous venous pulsation excludes raised intracranial pressure, but its absence does not necessarily confirm it, as 20% of normal subjects do not have spontaneous venous pulsation

Note: Papilloedema occurs as a result of interrupted axoplasmic flow in the optic nerve due to transmitted raised intracranial pressure. The manifestation is usually bilateral, but often with asymmetrical involvement of the optic nerve heads.

OPTIC NEURITIS

THE CRITERIA FOR OPTIC NEURITIS

- The patient is usually between 18 and under 45 years old
- Direct questioning will often reveal previous attacks in the same eye

- Optic neuritis may be bilateral but both eyes will not usually be affected simultaneously
- Periocular pain typically on moving the eye (present in 90% of cases)
- Significant visual loss within hours or a few days
- No further deterioration of vision after 7–10 days
- Afferent pupillary defect in the affected eye
- Colour vision defect in the affected eye
- Central or paracentral scotoma on the affected side
- Retrobulbar neuritis shows no changes in the optic nerve head (the patient sees nothing and the doctor sees nothing), whereas anterior neuritis (papillitis) usually presents with disc swelling. Optic atrophy may indicate a previous subclinical involvement but has to be considered with caution: neuro-imaging recommended
- Symptomatic improvement begins after 2–3 weeks

An atypical presentation of optic nerve neuritis is indication for CT imaging and haematological investigation.

TREATMENT AND MR IMAGING IN OPTIC NEURITIS

Commencement of treatment and MRI in a first attack of optic neuritis is left to the discretion of the doctor: a significant number of ophthalmologists will not treat or screen for multiple sclerosis in a first attack of optic neuritis.

Indication for commencement of treatment[1,2]	Optic nerve neuritis with two or more plaques of demyelination on MRI
Treatment[1,3]	1 g prednisolone i.v. daily[4], days 1–3
	1 mg/kg body weight orally daily, days 4–14
	20 mg, day 15
	10 mg, day 16
	No treatment on day 17
	10 mg, day 18

[1] Beck RW, Cleary P, Anderson MM *et al.* and the Optic Neuritis Study Group (1992) A randomized, controlled trial of corticosteroids in the treatment of acute optic neuritis. *N Engl J Med* **326**:581–588

[2] Contraindications include diabetes mellitus, cardiac disease, nephropathies, apoplexy

[3] Prior to the commencement of treatment, a systemic infection should be excluded (ESR, full blood count etc)

[4] The i.v. dose of prednisolone is given once daily in the morning in a 100 ml 0.9% NaCl solution or a 100 ml 5% glucose solution. During the three days of i.v. treatment, daily serum electrolytes and blood glucose checks should be performed and blood pressure checked

ISCHAEMIC OPTIC NEUROPATHY

DIAGNOSTIC CRITERIA

- The patient is usually over 45 years old; often diabetic or hypertensive
- Sudden and painless loss of vision
- Further deterioration of vision does not usually occur after the initial visual loss
- Rarely bilateral
- Nerve fibre bundle visual field defects may occur, most commonly inferior hemianopia
- Disc swelling may be partial or involve the whole optic nerve head. It resolves no later than 8 weeks after the onset of visual loss, and a segmental disc atrophy, corresponding to the visual field defect, may remain

Any unilateral disc swelling which does not comply with the above criteria requires CT/MRI imaging. Determination of ESR and C-reactive protein is often indicated, especially if the patient is over 65 years old and the visual loss is accompanied by periocular pain or preceded by headaches.

ARTERIOSCLEROTIC (NONARTERITIC) ANTERIOR ISCHAEMIC OPTIC NEUROPATHY (AION) VERSUS ARTERITIC AION

	Non-arteritic AION	Arteritic AION
Typical age (years)	60–65	70–75
Visual loss	Moderate to severe, sudden	Severe, sudden
Visual field	Inferior hemianopia; other nerve fibre bundle defects	Inferior hemianopia; central scotoma
Amaurosis fugax as an early sign	Rarely	Typical
Pain	None	Headaches and temporal tenderness, jaw claudication, polymyalgia rheumatica
Swollen optic nerve head	Yes	Yes (but sometimes no)
Disc size (compared with noninvolved eye)	Rather small	Any
Incidence	70%	30%
Prognosis for visual recovery	Usually slight improvement within a few months	Poor
Involvement of the other eye (without treatment)	Approximately $\frac{1}{3}$ of cases	Frequent
Occurrence of contralateral involvement	Months after the manifestation in the first eye	$\frac{1}{3}$ 1st day; $\frac{1}{3}$ 2nd day; $\frac{1}{3}$ 1st month; occurs rarely three days after commencement of systemic steroids

PSEUDOTUMOUR CEREBRI

CAUSES OF PSEUDOTUMOUR CEREBRI

Idiopathic	**Commonly seen in obese young females**	
Secondary	Cerebral or cavernous sinus thrombosis	
	Drugs	Tetracycline, penicillin, nalidixic acid, steroids, indomethacin, nitrofurantoin, vitamin A ($>25\,000$ IU)
	Endocrine	Hypoparathyroidism, adenocarcinoma of the adrenal glands
	Systemic disease	Lupus erythematosis, chronic respiratory insufficiency, iron deficiency anaemia

DIAGNOSIS OF PSEUDOTUMOUR CEREBRI

Symptoms	• Headaches, which get worse during Valsalva manoeuvre, are a common feature • Transient visual obscuration (TVO) • Visual field defects • Reduced visual acuity • Occasionally diplopia due to 6th nerve palsy
MRI	• No space-occupying mass • The ventricles are of normal size or small • Sometimes empty sella
CSF	• Increased intracranial pressure confirmed by lumbar puncture • Normal composition

TREATMENT OF PSEUDOTUMOUR CEREBRI

1. If possible treat the cause
2. Symptomatic
   Medical
      Weight loss
      Acetazolamide (high dosage needed)
      Steroids (for short periods of time only)
      Osmotics
   Invasive
      Repeated lumbar punctures
      Lumboperitoneal shunt
      Optic nerve decompression

CONGENITAL DISC ANOMALIES

Congenital disc anomalies

Large disc	Abnormal size of the optic nerve head, enlargement of the blind spot

Hypoplasia
Small disc, normal or reduced visual acuity.
De Morsier's syndrome (septo-optic dysplasia): short stature, nystagmus, optic disc hypoplasia, absent septum pellucidum. Early hormone substitution has good prognosis.

Coloboma
Dysplastic excavation usually situated inferonasally.
Morning glory syndrome: a rare dysplastic coloboma with sometimes other ocular and systemic associations (e.g. retinal detachment, persistent hyperplastic primary vitreous, absent corpus callosum, cleft palate).

Optic disc pit
Usually in the temporal part of the optic nerve head; dark grey appearance; serous detachment occurs not infrequently as a complication

Tilted disc syndrome
Often bilateral involvement; occasionally peripheral, bitemporal hemianopia, which is non-progressive and does not align with the vertical meridian as does a defect due to chiasmal disease; often associated with myopia and oblique astigmatism

Optic disc drüsen
Frequent cause of congenital disc swelling (in children, the drüsen are often deeply buried in the disc and not easily seen).
Typical signs:
• often absent disc cup or presence of a very small disc excavation
• autofluorescence (can be documented with red-free fundus photography)
• visual acuity usually remains unaffected
• visual field defects and peripapillary haemorrhages may occur; rarely, subretinal neovascular membranes
• nicely demonstrable with CT or ultrasound

Myelinated nerve fibres
Myelination of optic nerve fibres past the lamina cribrosa; clinical signs or complications do not occur

Bergmeister's papilla
Epi-papillary gliosis due to residual hyaloid artery

Haemangioma
Optic nerve haemangioma may be a manifestation of the von Hippel–Lindau syndrome

Pseudopapilloedema of hypermetropia
May occur in moderate or high hypermetropia

LOCALIZATION OF THE LESION IN VISUAL FIELD DEFECTS

TOPOGRAPHICAL DIAGNOSIS

Central scotoma	Optic neuropathy, optic nerve compression (the central fibres of the optic nerve are thin and least myelinated)
Caecocentral scotoma	Optic neuropathy Leber's optic neuropathy
Bjerrum's scotoma	Glaucoma, ischaemic optic neuropathy, juxtapapillary chorioretinitis
Superior or inferior hemi-anopia	Ischaemic optic neuropathy
Ipsilateral central scotoma with contralateral upper temporal defect (junction scotoma)	Lesion at the site where the optic nerve joins the chiasm (the contralateral superotemporal defect is caused by involvement of the anterior knee of Wilbrand)
Bitemporal hemianopia	Pituitary adenoma (enlargement of the sella turcica), but also meningioma, craniopharyngioma or aneurysm
Homonymous hemianopia	Lesion on the contralateral side, posterior to the chiasm
Incongruous homonymous hemianopia	Typically but not exclusively due to a lesion of the optic tract, sometimes of the lateral geniculate body (congruous homonymous hemianopia in lateral geniculate body lesions have also been reported)
Upper homonymous quadrantanopia ('pie in the sky')	Temporal lobe lesion (Meyer's loop)
Lower homonymous quadrantanopia	Parietal lobe lesion

OPTIC NERVE LESIONS VERSUS RETINAL VASCULAR LESIONS

Optic nerve lesions	Optic nerve lesions produce field loss with the apex at the fixation
Retinal vascular lesions	The retina is divided into quadrants by the vessels coming from the disc; consequently, retinal vascular lesions demonstrate field defects with the apex at the blind spot

LOCALIZATION OF THE LESION IN VISUAL FIELD DEFECTS

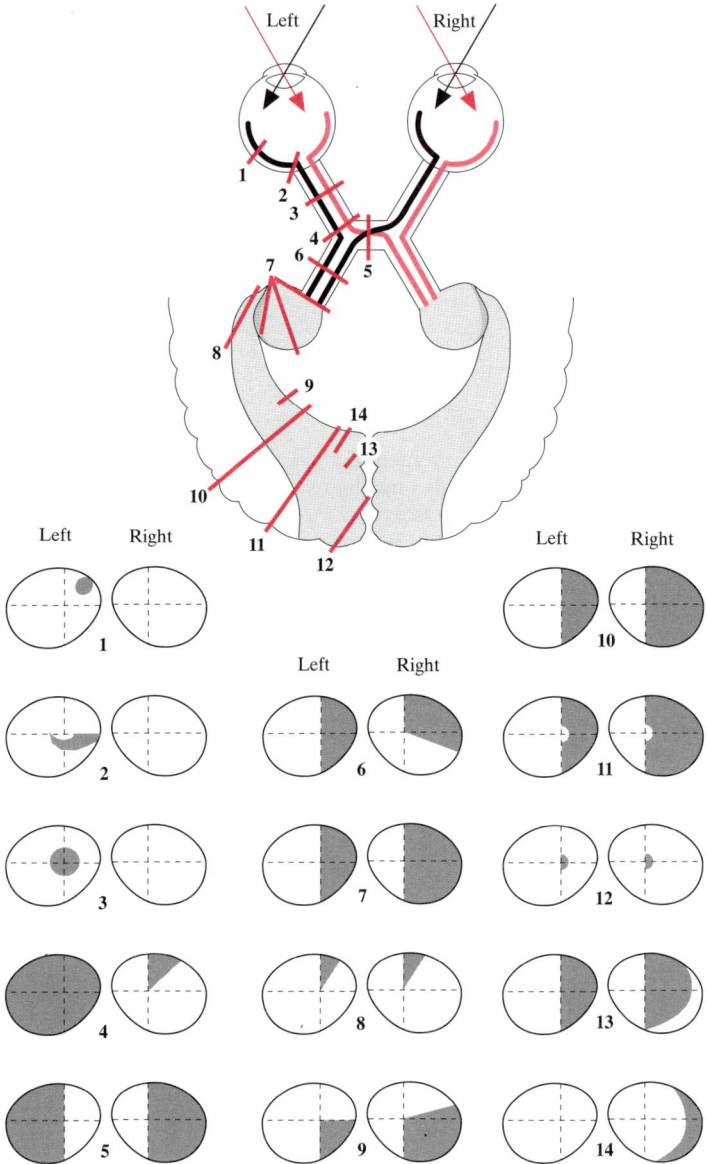

	Site of the lesion	Field defect
1	Retina	Variable; defects do not respect the vertical meridian
2	Nerve fibre bundle	Bjerrum's scotoma, enlarged blind spot, nasal step, etc.
3	Optic nerve	Centrocaecal or central scotomata
4	Optic nerve proximate to the chiasm and the anterior knee of Wilbrand	Ipsilateral central scotoma with contralateral upper temporal defect (junction scotoma)
5	Chiasm (decussating fibres)	Incomplete or full bitemporal hemianopia
6	Optic tract	Homonymous incomplete hemianopia with variable incongruity
7	Lateral geniculate body	Visual fields do not distinguish between lateral geniculate body lesions and lesions of the optic tract
8	Temporal lobe	Upper homonymous quadrantanopia (which always begin at the vertical meridian)
9	Parietal lobe	Lower homonymous quadrantanopia (other neurological defects such as agnosia or dysgraphia may coexist)
10	Visual cortex (anterior)	Homonymous congruous hemianopia
11	Visual cortex (posterior)	Homonymous congruous hemianopia with macular sparing
12	Occipital pole	Homonymous central or paracentral defects
13	Occipital lobe sparing the anterior calcarine	Homonymous hemianopia with contralateral crescent sparing
14	Anterior calcarine	Monocular contralateral crescent-shaped scotoma

VISUAL FIELDS IN CHIASM LESIONS

NERVE FIBRES WITHIN THE CHIASM

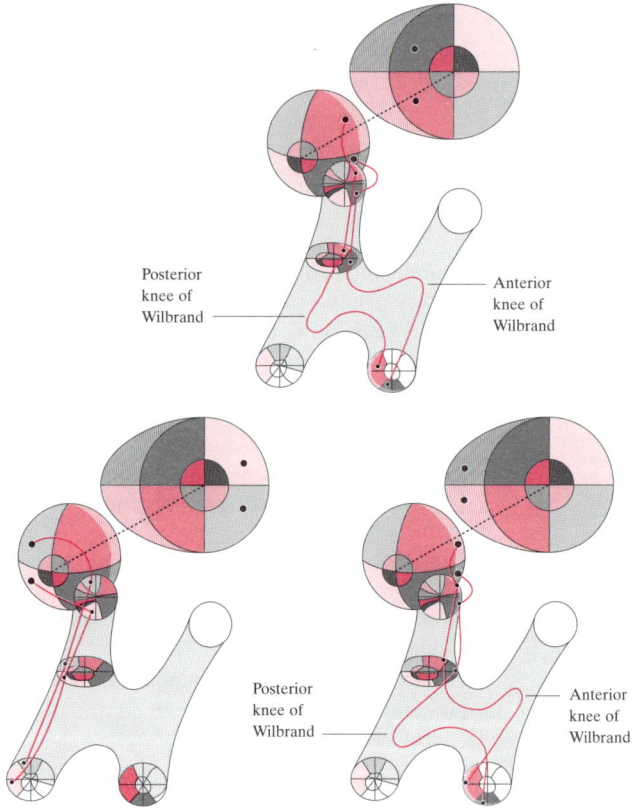

Posterior knee of Wilbrand

Anterior knee of Wilbrand

Posterior knee of Wilbrand

Anterior knee of Wilbrand

Visual field	Optic nerve	Chiasm	Optic tract
Central visual field	Laterally at the disc, then centrally	Mixture of crossed and uncrossed fibres	Upper and central parts of the tract
Nasal visual field	Lateral	Uncrossed	Superolateral
Temporal visual field	Medial	Crossed	Medial and inferior
Peripheral, superotemporal visual field	Medial	Anterior knee of Wilbrand	Medial and inferior
Peripheral, inferotemporal visual field	Medial	Posterior knee of Wilbrand	Medial and inferior

VISUAL FIELDS IN CHIASM LESIONS

Chiasmal compression	Common cause	Visual field defect	
Anterior–posteriorly or from below	Pituitary adenoma	Defects in the superotemporal quadrant; inferior extension in advanced cases	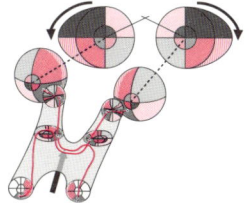
From superior and posterior	Craniopharyngeoma	Defects in the inferotemporal quadrant; superior extension in advanced cases	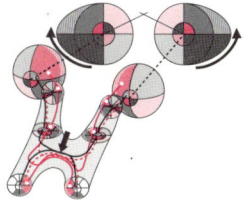
From laterally	Carotid aneurysm	Nasal visual field defects ipsilateral to the side of the lesion; binasal defects in advanced cases	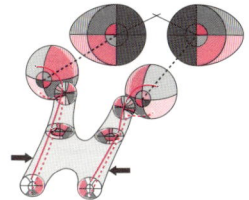
At the junction of optic nerve with chiasm		Ipsilateral central scotoma or temporal with contralateral upper temporal defect (the latter is caused by involvement of the anterior knee of Wilbrand)	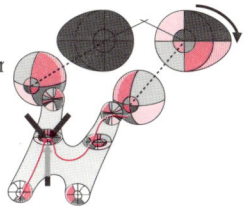
At the site where the optic tract leaves the chiasm		Homonymous incongruent defects with an inferotemporal defect, which is ipsilateral to the side of the lesion	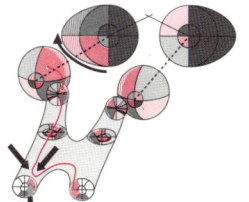

UNEXPLAINED VISUAL LOSS: DECISION-SUPPORTING ALGORITHM

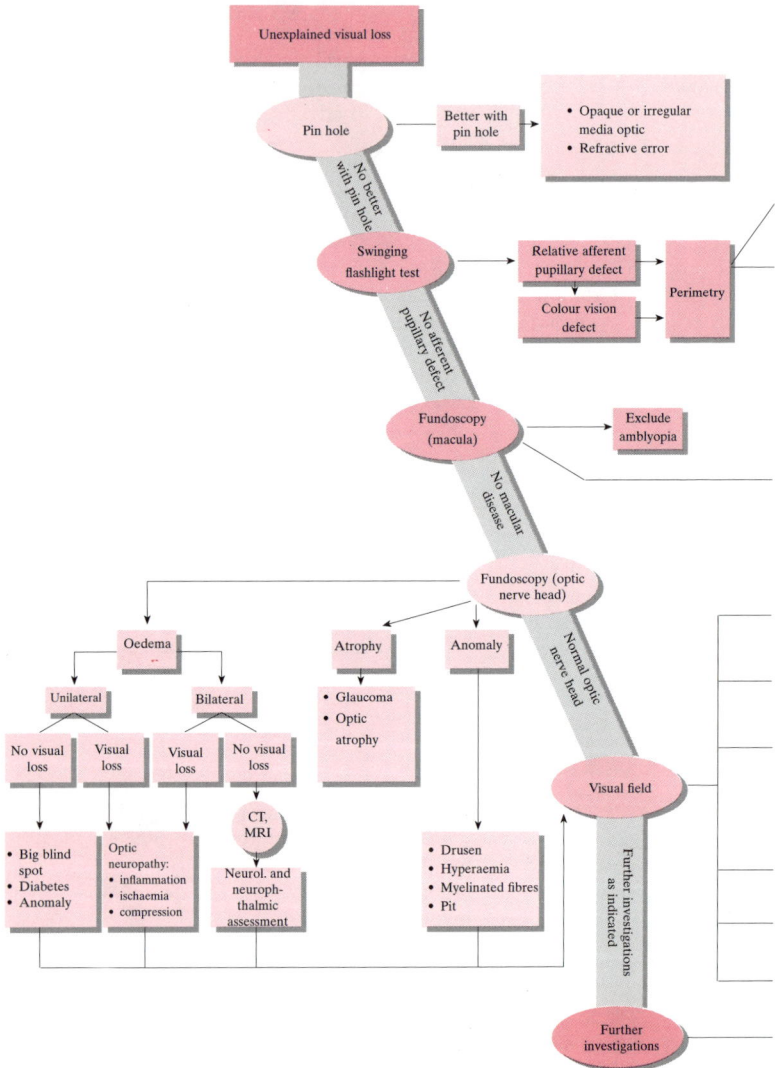

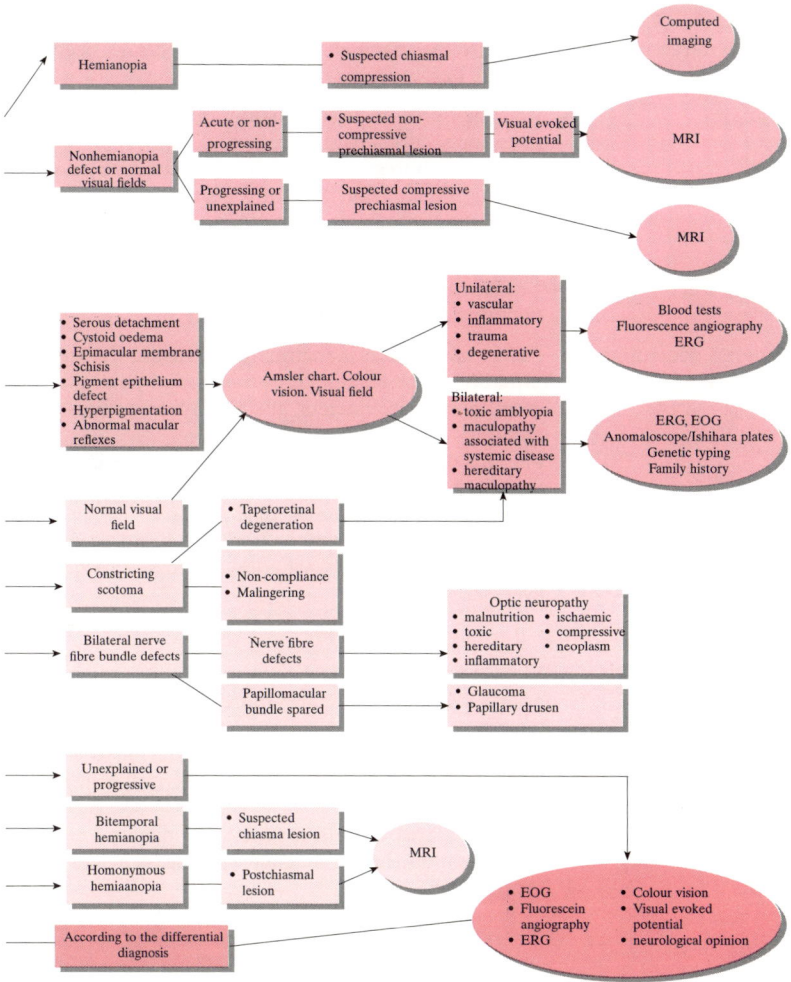

NOTES ON THE RETINAL REPRESENTATION WITHIN THE VISUAL PATHWAYS

Optic nerve	At the disc the macular fibres run temporally, becoming central 1 cm posterior to the disc
Chiasm	• Macular fibres decussate mainly in the superior and posterior sections of the chiasm • Inferonasal fibres loop into the opposite optic nerve forming the anterior knee of Wilbrand • Superonasal fibres loop into the ipsilateral optic tract (posterior knee of Wilbrand)
Optic tract	90° nasal rotation with the macular fibres running in the upper and central parts of the tract
Lateral geniculate body	• The nasal rotation is maintained, causing the superior retinal fibres to terminate in the medial part of the lateral geniculate nucleus and the inferior fibres to end laterally • The macular fibres account for most of the lateral geniculate nucleus with accurate correspondence of retinal points along the vertical axis • Crossed fibres terminate in layers 1, 4 and 6 of the lateral geniculate body, whereas uncrossed fibres end in layers 2, 3 and 5
Optic radiation	Nasal rotation is reversed
Visual cortex	• Accurate retinal–cortical correspondence (cortical lesions will therefore cause more congruous visual field defects) • The macula is projected over the posterior part of the visual cortex (hence central or paracentral scotomata in occipital pole lesions) • The foveal area of both maculae has bilateral cortical representation (hence macular sparing as a sign of occipital lobe lesions)

NOTES ON SUPRACHIASMAL LESIONS

Congruity	The more proximate the lesion is to the chiasm, the more incongruous the visual field defect
Foveal sparing	Sparing around fixation becomes significant with increasing distance to the chiasm (occipital lobe lesions typically cause homonymous hemianopia sparing the foveal area)

UNEXPLAINED VISUAL LOSS: WORK-UP

KEY STEPS FOR NARROWING DOWN THE DIFFERENTIAL DIAGNOSIS IN UNEXPLAINED VISUAL LOSS

Investigation	Result	Suspected diagnosis
Visual acuity with pin hole	Better	Optic media
Swinging flashlight test	Afferent pupillary defect	Prechiasmal or chiasmal lesion
Ophthalmoscopy	Dimished macular reflexes	Maculopathy
Ophthalmoscopy	Abnormal optic nerve head	Optic neuropathy
Visual field	Nerve fibre bundle defects	Optic neuropathy
Visual field	Incongruent defects, respecting the vertical meridian	Chiasmal lesion
Visual field	Homonymous hemianopia	Postchiasmal lesion
Visual field	Constriction	e.g. tapetoretinal degeneration
Amsler chart	Metamorphopsia	Maculopathy
History	Micropsia	Maculopathy
Colour vision	Abnormal	Cone dysfunction
Dark adaptation	Abnormal	Rod dysfunction
ERG, EOG, visual evoked potential	Abnormal	Dysfunction in various parts of the visual pathways
Fluorescence angiography	Abnormal (hyper- or hypofluorescence	An abnormal angiogram indicates retinal vascular malfunction or malfunction of the RPE

UNEXPLAINED VISUAL LOSS: FURTHER INVESTIGATIONS

RETINA, RETINAL PIGMENT EPITHELIUM, CHOROID

Suspected diagnosis	Investigation
Cone–rod dystrophy	ERG, EOG
Stargardt's disease	ERG, EOG, FFA, anomaloscope
X-linked juvenile retinoschisis	ERG
Toxic amblyopia	History, ERG, EOG, visual field
Tapetoretinal degeneration	EOG, ERG, dark adaptation, genetic typing
Retinal pigment epitheliopathy	EOG, fluorescence angiography, vitamin A, dark adaptation
Albinism	VER (determine ratio of decussating fibres)
Incomplete achromatopsia	Anomaloscope/Ishihara plates
Best's disease	EOG, fluorescence angiography
Central serous retinopathy	Fluorescence angiography, visual fields (static)

| Congenital stationary night blindness | Dark adaptation, ERG |
| Choroidal malcirculation | Indocyanine green angiography |

OPTIC NERVE HEAD

Suspected diagnosis	Investigation
Temporal arteritis	ESR, C-reactive protein, biopsy
Pseudotumour cerebri	CT
Leber's hereditary optic atrophy	Genetic typing
Optic neuritis	VECP (prolonged latency), afferent pupillary response, MRI
Ischaemic optic neuropathy	Blood pressure, afferent pupillary response, baseline blood tests
Autosomal dominant optic atrophy	Colour vision, check the family members
Posterior uveitis	Chest X-rays, blood tests

Chapter 11

BINOCULAR VISION/MOTILITY

The precondition for binocular vision is perception of the image simultaneously by both eyes (**simultaneous vision**). An ability to maintain a single fused image during vergence movements (**motor fusion**) is necessary to achieve binocular vision. The brain's ability to unite the images of both eyes into a single picture is called **sensory fusion**. The highest level of binocular vision is the ability of three-dimensional perception, called **stereopsis**.

The reference point for the main direction of vision is the fovea centralis. One point of the retina **corresponds** to an area of the other retina, **Panum's area**. The **horopter** is an area in space that corresponds to the exact point-for-point relationship of the retinal areas. **Panum's space** is the projection of Panum's area in space. **Stereopsis** occurs through deviation of the position of the visual object in front or behind the horopter within Panum's space. If Panum's area is transgressed, **physiological diplopia** occurs. The various fibres from Panum's area of a retina are connected, together with the fibres that correspond to the centre of the contralateral Panum's area, to one cortical neurone each.

Motor fusion fixes the nondominant eye on the centre of Panum's area, since here is the greatest number of synapses that project from both eyes to one cortical neurone.

Panum's areas have their greatest extension in the centre of the fovea centralis. If there is a small angle of squint, defects of fusion and of stereopsis occur or are primarily present. Fusion and binocular vision is still possible peripherally as long as the angle is not too large. In the sensitive phase (young children) double images in the centre of the visual field are suppressed (**suppression**). Deformation of Panum's areas displaces the peripheral spatial parameters. This deviation is transferred to the spatial parameter of the fovea ovalis of the squinting eye, the fovea centralis then no longer being the localizing centre of the squinting eye during binocular vision (**anomalous retinal correspondence, ARC**). In an extreme case this goes together with deviation of fixation in monocular vision to an eccentric retinal spot (extrafoveal fixation, **eccentric fixation**).

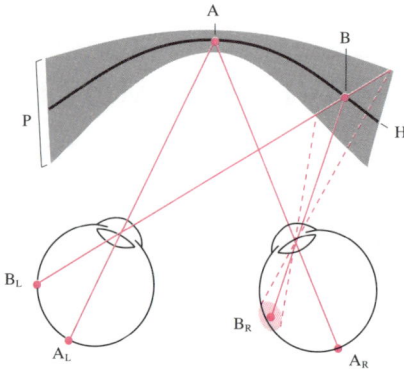

H   Horopter
P   Panum's fusional area
A'$_R$, A'$_L$ and B'$_R$, B'$_L$ are corresponding retinal points.
The Panum's area of B'$_R$ is indicated.

MOTILITY

INNERVATION OF THE EXTRAOCULAR MUSCLES

Nerve	Ipsilateral innervation	Contralateral innervation
Oculomotor nerve (III)		Superior rectus
	Medial rectus	
	Inferior rectus	
	Inferior oblique	
		Levator palpebrae
Trochlear nerve (IV)		Superior oblique
Abducens nerve (VI)	Lateral rectus	

NORMAL RANGE OF VERTICAL AND HORIZONTAL EYE MOVEMENTS

Abduction	45°	9–10 mm
Adduction	60°	9–10 mm
Elevation (supraduction, sursumduction)	50°	5–7 mm
Depression (infraduction, deorsumduction)	60°	9–10 mm

The range of ocular movements decreases in the elderly.

KESTENBAUM'S TEST

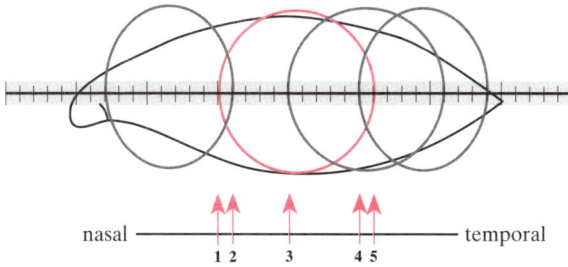

nasal ——————— temporal

1 2   3   4 5

Movement of the nasal limbus from position 1 to position 4 (9–10 mm)	Normal abduction
Movement of the nasal limbus from position 1 to position 3 (5 mm)	Reduced abduction
Movement of the temporal limbus from position 5 to position 2 (9–10 mm)	Normal adduction

The horizontal line represents a transparent ruler with millimetre marks.

FORMS OF EYE MOVEMENTS

Ductions **Monocular movements:** adduction, abduction, elevation, depression, incyclorotation, excyclorotation

Versions **Conjugate movements:** binocular synchronized eye movements in the same direction, e.g. dextroversion, laevoversion, supraversion, infraversion

Vergences **Disjugate movements:** binocular synchronized eye movements in opposite directions so that images of objects will fall on corresponding retinal points, e.g. convergence

THE NINE DIAGNOSTIC GAZE POSITIONS

Superior rectus muscle	Inferior oblique muscle	Superior rectus and inferior oblique muscles	Inferior oblique muscle	Superior rectus muscle
Lateral rectus muscle	Medial rectus muscle	Primary position	Medial rectus muscle	Lateral rectus muscle
Inferior oblique muscle	Superior oblique muscle	Inferior rectus muscle and superior oblique muscle	Superior oblique muscle	Inferior rectus muscle

INNERVATION LAWS OF OCULAR MOTILITY

Hering's Law   Yoke* agonist muscles and yoke antagonist muscles receive equal innervation

Sherrington's law of reciprocal innervation   Increased innervation of a contracting agonist muscle is accompanied by simultaneous decreased innervation of its antagonist

*Paired agonist muscles from each eye are referred to as yoke muscles

THE FUNCTION OF THE EXTRAOCULAR MUSCLES

	Primary	Secondary	Tertiary
Medial rectus	Adduction	–	–
Lateral rectus	Abduction	–	–
Superior rectus	Elevation	Adduction	Incyclorotation
Inferior rectus	Depression	Adduction	Excyclorotation
Superior oblique	Incyclorotation	Depression	Abduction
Inferior oblique	Excyclorotation	Elevation	Abduction

Note: The upper muscles (superior rectus and superior oblique) are incyclorotators, the lower muscles (inferior rectus and inferior oblique) are excyclorotators.

DIAGRAM SHOWING THE FUNCTION OF THE EXTRA-OCULAR MUSCLES

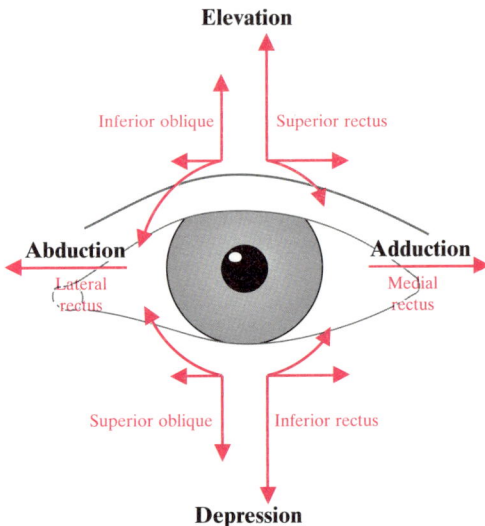

SYNERGISTIC FUNCTIONS OF THE VERTICAL CONTRIBUTORS

Elevation	Superior rectus	Inferior oblique
Depression	Inferior rectus	Superior oblique
Incyclorotation	Superior oblique	Superior rectus
Excyclorotation	Inferior oblique	Inferior rectus
Adduction (medial rectus)	Superior rectus	Inferior rectus
Abduction (lateral rectus)	Superior oblique	Inferior oblique

CONCOMITANT STRABISMUS DIVIDED ACCORDING TO THE POSITION OF THE DEVIATING EYE

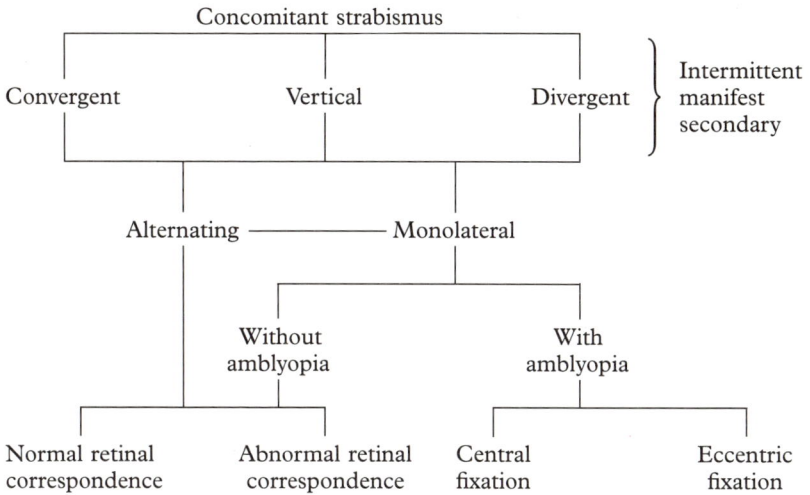

PSEUDOSTRABISMUS

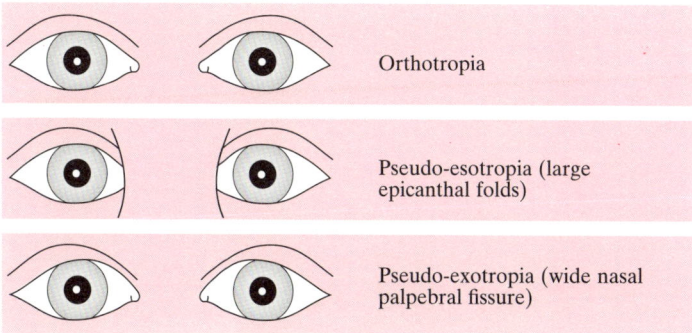

Orthotropia

Pseudo-esotropia (large epicanthal folds)

Pseudo-exotropia (wide nasal palpebral fissure)

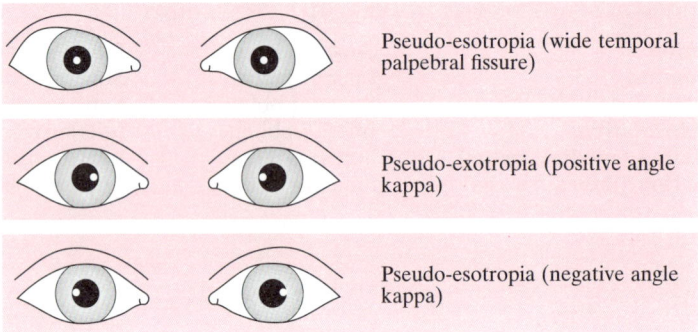

Pseudo-esotropia (wide temporal palpebral fissure)

Pseudo-exotropia (positive angle kappa)

Pseudo-esotropia (negative angle kappa)

OCULAR AXES AND ANGLES

Angle alpha (α)   Angle between optical and anatomical axes
Angle gamma (γ)   Angle between optical and visual axes
Angle kappa (ϰ)   Angle between anatomical and visual axes

ESTIMATION OF OCULAR DEVIATION

HIRSCHBERG TEST

(a corneal light reflex test for estimation of ocular deviation)

Ocular deviation

Light reflex displacement of 1 mm	**7°**
Light reflex on pupillary margin (4 mm pupillary diameter)	**+15°**
Light reflex on temporal limbus	**+40°**
Light reflex on nasal limbus	**−35°**

RETINAL CORRESPONDENCE

INTERPRETATION OF THE AFTERIMAGE TEST IN PATIENTS WITH CENTRAL FIXATION

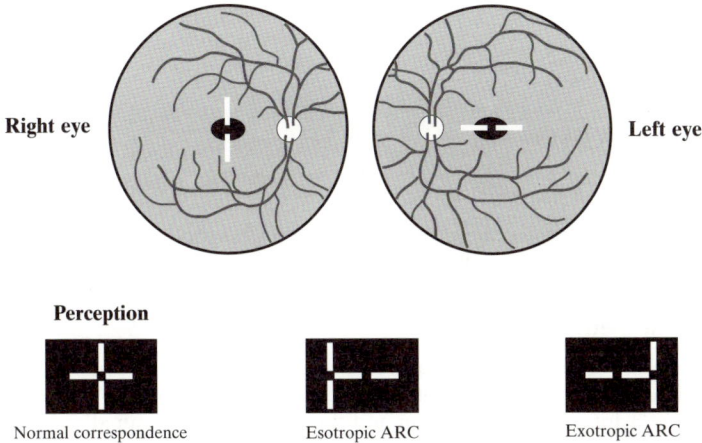

Right eye   Left eye

Perception

Normal correspondence   Esotropic ARC   Exotropic ARC

AMBLYOSCOPE READINGS

Subjective angle	The amount in degrees that the examiner must move the amblyoscopic arms to allow the patient to see the two pictures as being superimposed
Objective angle	In contrast to the subjective angle, the objective angle is measured under alternating monocular viewing. It equals the deviation as measured by the alternate prism cover test

RETINAL CORRESPONDENCE

Normal retinal correspondence (NRC)	The two foveas have no different visual directions Subjective angle = objective angle; angle of anomaly = 0
Harmonious anomalous retinal correspondence (HARC)	The fovea of the fixating eye acquires an anomalous common visual direction with a periphereal area in the retina of the deviated eye Subjective angle = 0; angle of anomaly = objective angle
Disharmonious anomalous retinal correspondence (DARC)	The amount of the shift in visual directions does not fully compensate for the deviation Subjective angle ≠ 0; angle of anomaly ≠ objective angle

STEREO-ACUITY

IMAGE DISPARITY OF THE TITMUS TEST IN SECONDS OF ARC

Fly	3800″		
Animals	A 400″	B 200″	C 100″
Circles	1.800″	2.400″	3.200″
	4.140″	5.100″	6.80″
	7.60″	8.50″	9.40″

AC/A RATIO

MEASURING THE AC/A RATIO

The AC/A ratio is the amount of change in convergence (AC; cm/m) for a specific amount of change in accommodation (A; dpt).

Gradient method

The amount of deviation is measured with full correction at distance using an accommodative target. A -3 dpt lens is then placed in front of both eyes to stimulate 3 dpt of accommodation and the deviation remeasured.

$$\text{AC/A} = \frac{\text{deviation with added} -3.0 \text{ sphere} - \text{deviation with full correction}}{3}$$

Example

Distance deviation without supplement = +45
Distance deviation with +3.0 lens = +15

$$\text{AC/A} = \frac{45 - 15}{3} = 10 \left(\text{high}\right)$$

Heterophoria method

The heterophoria method compares the deviation in the distance and near range to determine the AC/A ratio. The distance and near deviation is measured in prism dpt, the interpupillary distance in cm.

D = distance deviation (prism dpt)
N = near deviation (prism dpt)
IPD = interpupillary distance (cm)
DA = dioptres of accommodation for near fixation ($^1/_3$ m = 3 dpt)

$$\text{AC/A} = IPD + \frac{N - D}{DA}$$

Example

D = +42 prism dpt
N = +33 prism dpt at $^1/_3$ m

IPD = 6 cm
DA = 3 dpt

$$AC/A = 6 + \frac{42 - 33}{3} = 9 \left(\text{high}\right)$$

BAGOLINI STRIATED LENSES

INTERPRETATION OF THE BAGOLINI LENSES TEST

Perception	Orthotropia	Heterotropia
Two lines crossing at the centre 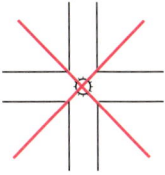	Normale retinal correspondence	Harmonious ARC
One line 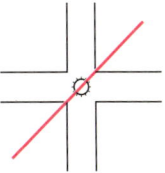	Suppression	Suppression
Two lines, one with a gap centrally 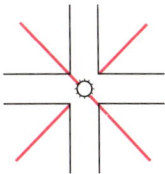	Central scotoma, e.g. in anisometropia	Microtropia (small central scotoma, peripheral fusion, fixation point with harmonious ARC)
Two lines, one displaced 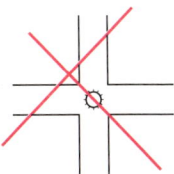		NRC or disharmonious ARC

FIXATION

CATEGORIES OF FIXATION

1. Foveolar fixation
2. Parafoveolar fixation
3. Parafoveal fixation
4. Peripheral fixation
5. No fixation

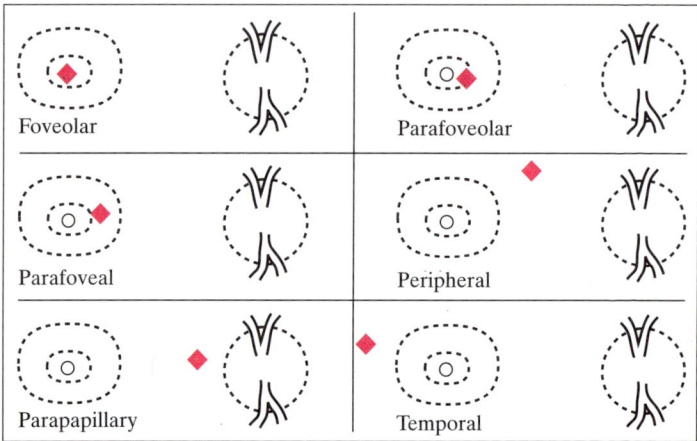

RELATIONSHIP BETWEEN THE VISUAL ACUITY AND POINT OF FIXATION

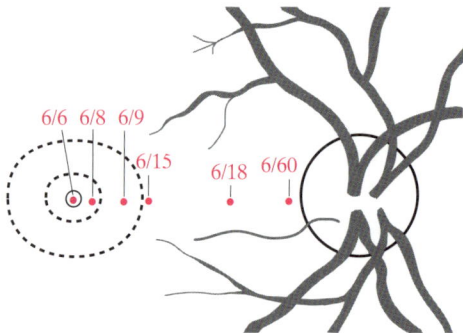

AMBLYOPIA/MICROSTRABISMUS

FIXATION BEHAVIOUR OF THE AFFECTED EYE IN
PRIMARY MICROSTRABISMUS

• **(1) Microstrabismus with central fixation:** there is ARC, but no eccentric
fixation [ARC]

- **(2) Microstrabismus with eccentric fixation:** neither the central reference point of ARC, nor the area of eccentric fixation are identical.
- **(3) Microstrabismus with identity:** the central point of ARC and the area of eccentric fixation are identical. Cover/uncover tests reveal no manifest strabismus.

TYPES OF AMBLYOPIA

Type	Cause	Example
Strabismus amblyopia	Suppression	Microstrabismus
Anisometropic amblyopia	Suppression, deprivation due to a marked disparity in the refractive error	Anisohyperopia
Deprivation amblyopia	Deprivation of visual stimulus	Haemangioma, congenital cataract
Organic amblyopia	Damage to the foveal receptors at birth or early childhood	Toxoplasmosis infection causing macular lesion
Bilateral amblyopia	Bilateral maldevelopment of visual maturation due to blurred retinal images in both eyes	Congenital nystagmus

AMBLYOPIGENIC FACTORS

1. Deprivation
   - bilateral deprivation (e.g. cataract)
   - marked ametropia
   - nystagmus
2. Deprivation and abnormal biocular interactions (suppression)
   - anisometropia
   - monocular deprivation (e.g. cataract, ptosis)

SEVERITY OF AMBLYOPIA

Visual acuity	Severity
6/60 or less	Severe
6/12 or less	Moderate
6/9 or less	Mild

TREATMENT OF AMBLYOPIA

(n = age of the patient in years)

I.   Bilateral normal vision, bilateral central fixation and alternating strabismus:
     No occlusion
     three monthly follow-ups

II. Bilateral normal vision, bilateral central fixation and monolateral strabismus:

Intermittent patching or penalization of the dominant eye

III. Unilateral amblyopia, bilateral central fixation:

Intermittent occlusion (at least two days per week or four hours a day); with visual acuity <0.8: *n* days per week occlusion of the dominant eye and one day without occlusion

IV. Extrafoveal fixation:

Continuous patching over *n* days with subsequent follow-up:

1. If the examination shows central fixation, continue as III
2. If, on examination, the fixation remains noncentral, but has improved, continue occlusion of the dominant eye over 3 × *n* days with subsequent follow-up
3. If visual acuity remains unchanged or fixation becomes more peripheral, try inverse occlusion (i.e. occlusion of the nondominant eye) over *n* days with subsequent follow-up:
   • If improvement on examination, retry occlusion of the dominant eye
   • If no improvement, retry inverse occlusion with following occlusion of the dominant eye

Notes: Occlusion of the dominant eye should be discontinued if the follow-up examination shows diminution of the ipsilateral visual acuity

INFANTILE ESOTROPIA

CLINICAL FEATURES AND ASSOCIATED MOTOR ABNORMALITIES OF ESSENTIAL INFANTILE ESOTROPIA

Large convergent angle	Infantile esotropia is usually a large-angle constant esotropia. Some cases show variable angle, independent of accomodation
Latent nystagmus	Occlusion of one eye leads to a jerk nystagmus with the fast component away from the covered eye
Dissociated vertical deviation (DVD)	A slow upward turn of the nonfixating (covered) eye. The alternate cover test reveals that each eye turns upward under cover in contrast to the response in vertical, heterophoria
Gaze-dependent ocular alignment	A-pattern: reduced convergence in down gaze V-pattern: decreased esodeviation in up gaze. Most frequently associated with inferior oblique overaction and superior oblique underfunction
Abnormal head posture	A face turn to the side of the dominant eye is typical. A head tilt to the same side may coexist
Cyclorotation	Usually an incyclorotation of the eye that takes up fixation, whereas the other eye (that gives up fixation) does an upward turn and an excyclorotation

Age	Severity of amblyopia	Occlusion	Follow-up
<3 months	Any	Nil	At 4 months of age
3–12 months	Any	Dominant eye; 1 hour daily, up to half of the waking time	Monthly
12–24 months	Mild	Dominant eye; 4 hours daily	Monthly
	Moderate	Dominant eye; half of the waking time	
	Severe	Dominant eye all day, and both eyes unoccluded every other day	

ABNORMAL HEAD POSTURE (OCULAR TOR-ICOLLIS)

AN OCULAR CAUSE FOR AN ABNORMAL HEAD POSTURE IS LIKELY, IF

1. it becomes more obvious when the patient observes targets which need good acuity
2. it does not persist during sleep
3. it resolves in occlusion

ABNORMAL HEAD POSTURE DUE TO FALSE CYLINDER AXIS (IN HIGH ASTIGMATISM)

The lens is to be turned in the direction of the abnormal head posture. For example, a given cylinder axis of 90° (where the needed cylinder axis is 100°) may lead to a head tilt to the right shoulder.

CAUSES OF NYSTAGMUS ASSOCIATED ABNORMAL HEAD POSTURE

- A jerk nystagmus with a null point outside the primary position
- Decreased nystagmus in convergence
- Preservation of binocular vision in latent nystagmus with coexisting motility disorder
- Decreased nystagmus due to mechanical restriction in the end-gaze position

ABNORMAL HEAD POSTURE DUE TO RESTRICTED OCULAR MOTILITY

Affected muscle (restricted action)	Acquired head posture
Lateral rectus (restricted abduction)	Face turn to the affected side
Superior rectus (restricted up-gaze, especially in abduction)	Chin elevation and face turn to the affected side

Affected muscle (restricted action)

Inferior rectus (restricted down-gaze in abduction)

Superior oblique (restricted intorsion, restricted depression)

Bilateral superior oblique

Inferior oblique (restricted extorsion, restricted elevation)

Acquired head posture

Chin depression and face turn to the affected side

Head tilt and face turn to the opposite side, chin depression

Chin depression

Head tilt and face turn to the affected side, chin elevation

ASTHENOPIA

CAUSES OF ASTHENOPIA ('EYE STRAIN')

Functional

Ametropia with unsuited correction
Accommodation malfunction
Heterophoria
Convergence malfunction
Fusion insufficiency
Anisometropia, aniseikonia
Decompensated microtropia

Organic

Opaque media
Graves' ophthalmopathy
Iritis, iridocyclitis
Glaucoma
Maculopathies

Neurological

Acquired nystagmus
Tonic pupil
Superior oblique myokymia
Migraine
Intracranial pressure
Cervical headache
Psychogenic

NORMAL FUSIONAL RESERVES

Fusional convergence	~40 cm/m (15–25°)
Fusional divergence	~10 cm/m (4–6°)
Vertical fusion	~5 cm/m (3–6°)
Cyclofusion	0–20°

Note: Divergence fusional reserves are measured using base-in prisms with increased power over one eye until the patient reaches the blur point. Convergence reserves are measured similarly using base-out prisms. Vertical reserves are measured by placing base-down prisms in front of the right eye or base-up prisms in front of the left eye (positive), base-up prisms in front of the right eye or base-down prisms in front of the left eye and base-up in front of the left eye (negative).

PRISM THERAPY

INDICATION FOR PRESCRIPTION OF PRISMS

Heterophoria with asthenopia	Up to 10 prism dioptres (PD) usually tolerable; long-term satisfactory results often achievable in eso- and verticophoria, more infrequently achieved in exophoria
Moderate paresis with diplopia in primary position	Up to 30 prism dioptres (PD); Frequent follow-ups are recommended, because spontaneous recovery of the paretic muscle (common in diabetes mellitus and hypertension) may require adjustment of prism.
Late onset of diplopia in manifest concomitant strabismus	Prism is prescribed to enable the 're-use' of the adapted suppression scotoma and is therefore to be placed over the non-dominant (non-fixing) eye
Decompensated microesotropia	The given prism should neutralize the subjective (not the objective) angle; placing the prism over the dominant eye as an occlusion therapy may be considered; early surgical correction is desirable
Normosensory late onset heterotropia (diploplia usually indicates acquired strabismus with onset after five years of age)	Prism therapy indicated until surgery

Note:
- Ocular misalignment may be measured in degrees or prism dioptres (PD). The power of a prism in PD (Δ) is equal to the shift, in cm, of a light-ray passing through the prism, measured 1 m from the prism: 1 PD desplaces a light-ray 1 cm at 1 m from the prism.
- When converting PD to degrees, 1° is equal to 2Δ. This is roughly correct for small angles. Beyond 45° (100Δ), the number of PD per degree increases exponentially: degrees = $\tan^1 (\Delta/100)$.
- Fresnel press-on prisms decrease the visual acuity by approximately 3% per PD.

CONVERTING PD INTO DEGREES IN EMMETROPIA AND IN REFRACTIVE ERROR WITH OPTICAL CORRECTION

Prism dioptres	Refraction	Angle of deviation
10Δ	0 dpt	6°
10Δ	+10 dpt	8°
10Δ	−10 dpt	5°
25Δ	0 dpt	13°
25Δ	+10 dpt	18°
25Δ	−10 dpt	10°
40Δ	0 dpt	18°

Prism dioptres	Refraction	Angle of deviation
40Δ	+10 dpt	25°
40Δ	−10 dpt	14°

Note: Glasses produce a prismatic change of the deviation as measured in front of the glasses. Minus lenses increase the measured angle of deviation whilst plus lenses decrease the measured angle. This becomes clinically significant in optical corrections of more than +5 dpt or less than −5 dpt.

PRISM NOMOGRAPH FOR DETERMINING THE OBLIQUE PRISM

For example

A vertical prism of 4 cm/m base 90° and a horizontal prism of 7 cm/m base 0° results in an oblique prism of approx. 8 cm/m base 30°.

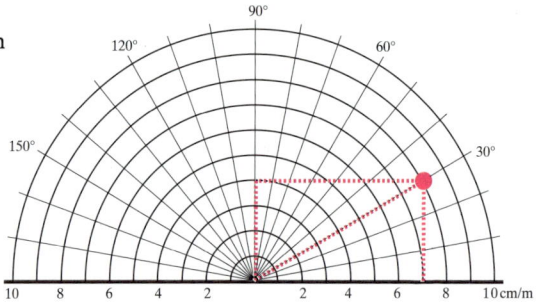

TABLE FOR DETERMINING OBLIQUE PRISMS

[cm/m = Δ]	Base position 0° 1	2	3	4	5	6	7	8	9	10
1	1.4Δ 45°	2.2Δ 27°	3.2Δ 18°	4.1Δ 14°	5.1Δ 11°	6.1Δ 9°	7.1Δ 8°	8.1Δ 7°	9.1Δ 6°	10Δ 6°
2	2.2Δ 63°	2.8Δ 45°	3.6Δ 34°	4.5Δ 27°	5.4Δ 22°	6.3Δ 18°	7.3Δ 16°	8.2Δ 14°	9.2Δ 12°	10.2Δ 11°
3	3.2Δ 72°	3.6Δ 56°	4.2Δ 45°	5.0Δ 37°	5.8Δ 32°	6.7Δ 27°	7.6Δ 23°	8.5Δ 21°	9.5Δ 18°	10.4Δ 17°
4	4.1Δ 76°	4.5Δ 63°	5.0Δ 53°	5.7Δ 45°	6.4Δ 39°	7.2Δ 34°	8.1Δ 30°	8.9Δ 27°	9.8Δ 24°	10.8Δ 22°
5	5.1Δ 79°	5.4Δ 68°	5.8Δ 59°	6.4Δ 51°	7.1Δ 45°	7.8Δ 40°	8.6Δ 35°	9.4Δ 32°	10.3Δ 29°	11.2Δ 27°
6	6.1Δ 81°	6.3Δ 72°	6.7Δ 63°	7.2Δ 56°	7.8Δ 50°	8.5Δ 45°	9.2Δ 41°	10.0Δ 37°	11.0Δ 34°	11.7Δ 31°
7	7.1Δ 82°	7.3Δ 74°	7.6Δ 67°	8.1Δ 60°	8.6Δ 55°	9.2Δ 49°	9.9Δ 45°	10.6Δ 41°	11.4Δ 38°	12.2Δ 35°
8	8.1Δ 83°	8.2Δ 76°	8.5Δ 69°	9.0Δ 63°	9.4Δ 58°	10.0Δ 53°	10.6Δ 49°	11.3Δ 45°	12.0Δ 42°	12.8Δ 39°
9	9.1Δ 84°	9.2Δ 78°	9.5Δ 72°	9.8Δ 66°	10.3Δ 61°	10.8Δ 56°	11.4Δ 52°	12.0Δ 48°	12.7Δ 45°	13.5Δ 42°
10	10.0Δ 84°	10.2Δ 79°	10.4Δ 73°	10.8Δ 68°	11.2Δ 63°	11.7Δ 59°	12.2Δ 55°	12.8Δ 51°	13.5Δ 48°	14.1Δ 45°

Base position 90°

For example:
Prisms add as ordinary vectors. A horizontal prism of 4 cm/m (Δ) base 0°
combined with a vertical prism of 3 cm/m (Δ) base 90° will be prescribed as
a single oblique prism of 5 cm/m (Δ) base 37°.

Note: The power of an oblique prism can also be determined by drawing a
triangle: the first two sides of the triangle are proportional to the measured
horizontal and vertical prisms and are placed at 90° to each other. The third
side is proportional to the amount of oblique prism needed. The orientation
of the prism base is determined by measuring the appropriate angle with
a protractor on a trial frame.

SQUINT SURGERY

Distance of muscle insertion from the limbus	Maximal recession and resection of the extraocular muscles in squint surgery: guidelines to avoid post-operative incomitance	
Medial rectus: 5.5 mm	Recession 5 mm	Resection 6 mm
Lateral rectus: 7.5 mm	Recession 8 mm	Resection 8 mm
Inferior rectus: 6.5 mm	Recession 6 mm	Resection 6 mm
Superior rectus: 8 mm	Recession 6 mm	Resection 6 mm
Superior oblique: 14–16 mm	Recession 8 mm	Tuck 5–8 mm (age-dependent)
Inferior oblique: 18 mm	Recession 10 mm	Resection 4 mm

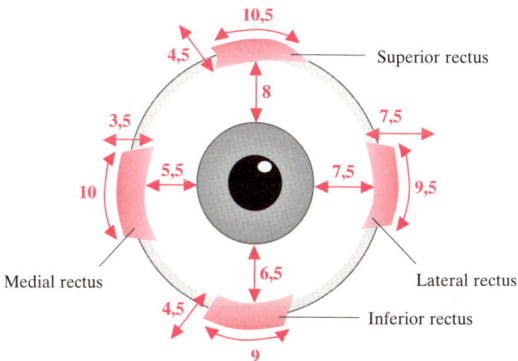

The distance from the limbus, insertion width and tendon length are
indicated

HORIZONTAL RECTUS MUSCLE TRANSPOSITION FOR A- AND V-PATTERNS

Pattern	Medial rectus transposition	Lateral rectus transposition
V-patterns	Down	Up
A-patterns	Up	Down

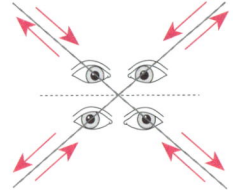

Note: The muscles are transposed in the direction in which their horizontal motor function is to be weakened.

DIPLOPIA: EXAMINATION

THE TWO COMPONENTS OF DOUBLE VISION

Diplopia The same image is seen in two different locations
Confusion Two different images are seen superimposed on top of each other

Note: Acquired strabismus in older children or adults usually causes diplopia. Confusion is less common than diplopia and tends to occur in patients with acquired strabismus and restricted visual fields forcing the simultaneous use of both foveas.

IMAGE LOCATION IN DIPLOPIA

Type of deviation	Perceived diplopia
Convergent strabismus	Uncrossed
Divergent strabismus	Crossed
Positive vertical strabismus (right over left)	The image of the right eye is seen below the image of the left eye
Negative vertical strabismus (left over right)	The image of the right eye is seen above the image of the left eye
Excyclotropia	Inward tilt of the diplopia
Incyclotropia	Outward tilt of the diplopia

Location of diplopic images ⇒ shifted to the opposite side of the deviation
Distance between the double images ⇒ proportional to the angle of the deviation

THE RED GLASS TEST

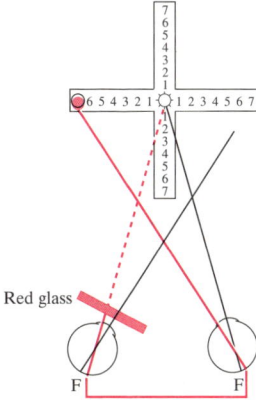

Red glass test in convergent strabismus:

Homonymous or uncrossed diplopia The right eye fixates on the white light. In the left eye, the red light falls on a nasal retinal area which corresponds to a temporal retinal area in the right eye. The red light is seen left of the white light.

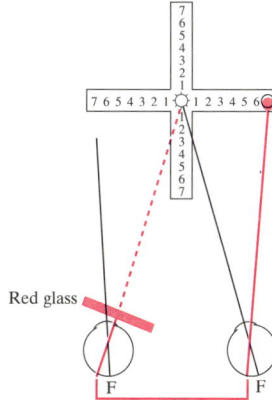

Red glass test in divergent strabismus:

Heteronymous or crossed diplopia The right eye fixates on the white light. In the left eye, the red light falls on a temporal retinal area which corresponds to a nasal retinal area in the right eye. The red light is seen right of the white light.

DIPLOPIA: DIAGNOSTIC PATHWAY

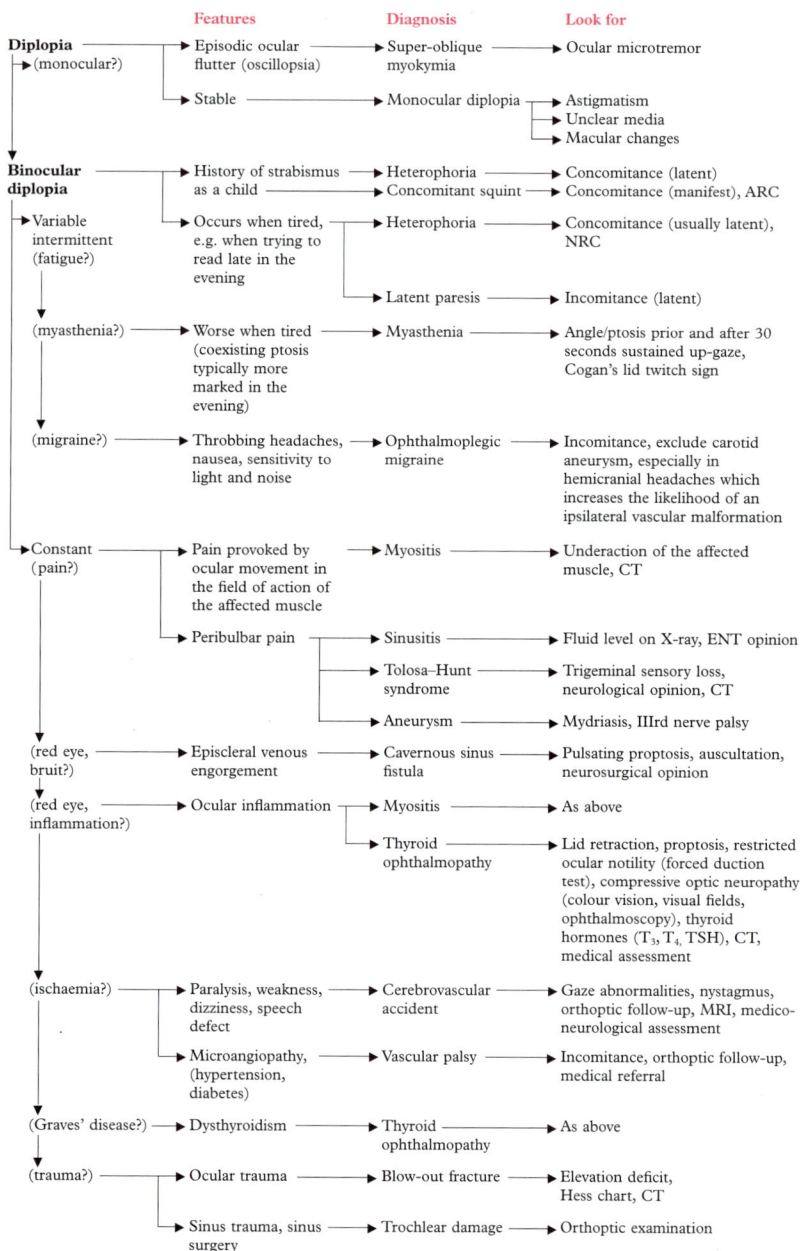

	Features	Diagnosis	Look for

Diplopia → (monocular?) → Episodic ocular flutter (oscillopsia) → Super-oblique myokymia → Ocular microtremor

→ Stable → Monocular diplopia → Astigmatism / Unclear media / Macular changes

Binocular diplopia

→ History of strabismus as a child → Heterophoria → Concomitance (latent)
→ Concomitant squint → Concomitance (manifest), ARC

→ Variable intermittent (fatigue?) → Occurs when tired, e.g. when trying to read late in the evening → Heterophoria → Concomitance (usually latent), NRC

→ Latent paresis → Incomitance (latent)

(myasthenia?) → Worse when tired (coexisting ptosis typically more marked in the evening) → Myasthenia → Angle/ptosis prior and after 30 seconds sustained up-gaze, Cogan's lid twitch sign

(migraine?) → Throbbing headaches, nausea, sensitivity to light and noise → Ophthalmoplegic migraine → Incomitance, exclude carotid aneurysm, especially in hemicranial headaches which increases the likelihood of an ipsilateral vascular malformation

→ Constant (pain?) → Pain provoked by ocular movement in the field of action of the affected muscle → Myositis → Underaction of the affected muscle, CT

→ Peribulbar pain → Sinusitis → Fluid level on X-ray, ENT opinion
→ Tolosa–Hunt syndrome → Trigeminal sensory loss, neurological opinion, CT
→ Aneurysm → Mydriasis, IIIrd nerve palsy

(red eye, bruit?) → Episcleral venous engorgement → Cavernous sinus fistula → Pulsating proptosis, auscultation, neurosurgical opinion

(red eye, inflammation?) → Ocular inflammation → Myositis → As above
→ Thyroid ophthalmopathy → Lid retraction, proptosis, restricted ocular notility (forced duction test), compressive optic neuropathy (colour vision, visual fields, ophthalmoscopy), thyroid hormones (T_3, T_4, TSH), CT, medical assessment

(ischaemia?) → Paralysis, weakness, dizziness, speech defect → Cerebrovascular accident → Gaze abnormalities, nystagmus, orthoptic follow-up, MRI, medico-neurological assessment

→ Microangiopathy, (hypertension, diabetes) → Vascular palsy → Incomitance, orthoptic follow-up, medical referral

(Graves' disease?) → Dysthyroidism → Thyroid ophthalmopathy → As above

(trauma?) → Ocular trauma → Blow-out fracture → Elevation deficit, Hess chart, CT

→ Sinus trauma, sinus surgery → Trochlear damage → Orthoptic examination

THE CRANIAL NERVES AND THEIR FUNCTION

Cranial nerve	somatomotor	branchiomotor	visceromotor	viscerosensory	somatosensory	sensory	Function
I Olfactory						•	Sense of smell
II Optic						•	Vision
III Oculomotor	•						All external occular muscles except the superior oblique and lateral rectus
			•				Ciliary muscle, sphincter pupillae
IV Trochlear	•						Superior oblique
V Trigeminal	•						Mastication (V_3)
					•		Face, nose, teeth, mouth
VI Abducens	•						Lateral rectus
VII Facial		•					Facial expression muscles, platysma, tensor tympani
			•				Lacrimal glands, submaxillary glands, sublingual glands
					•		Parts of the ear
						•	Taste (from anterior two-thirds of tongue)
VIII Vestibulocochlear						•	Equilibrium and orientation of the body in space (vestibular nerve), sense of hearing (cochlear nerve)
IX Glossopharyngeal		•					Swallowing
			•				Parotid glands
				•			Carotid sinus
					•		Oral and pharyngeal sensations
						•	Taste (posterior third of tongue)
X Vagus		•					Pharyngeal and laryngeal muscles
			•				Smooth muscles and glands of pharynx and larynx
				•			Pharynx, larynx, thoracic and abdominal viscera
					•		Pharynx, larynx, thoracic and abdominal viscera
XI Accessory	•						Sternocleidomastoid muscle, trapezius muscle
XII Hypoglossal	•						Movements of the tongue

ABDUCENS NERVE PALSY

SITES OF LESION AND CAUSES OF ABDUCENS NERVE PALSY

Orbit

exophthalmos and various combinations with palsies of the IIIrd and IVth nerves may occur
- posterior orbit tumour (orbital apex syndrome)
- pseudotumour of the orbit
- thyroid disease
- orbital cellulitis

Superior orbital fissure, cavernous sinus

sympathetic plexus lesion and palsies of the III, IV and V nerves may coexist
- intracavernous internal carotid artery aneurysm
- carotid cavernous sinus fistula
- nasopharyngeal malignancy (Godtfredsen's syndrome)
- sphenoidal sinusitis
- Tolosa–Hunt syndrome

Skull base and brain stem

- cerebellopontine angle tumour
- increased intracranial pressure, pseudotumour cerebri
- craniocerebral trauma
- Gradenigo's syndrome
- inflammation (multiple sclerosis)
- pontine lesions: may involve the lateral gaze centre resulting in loss of conjugate lateral gaze towards the side of the lesion. Contralateral hemiplegia and Vth nerve involvement (ipsilateral loss of facial sensation) may coexist

Systemic, non-localized

- diabetic neuropathy
- infectious
- toxic (e.g. Wernicke–Korsakoff syndrome)

CAVERNOUS SINUS AND SUPERIOR ORBITAL FISSURE

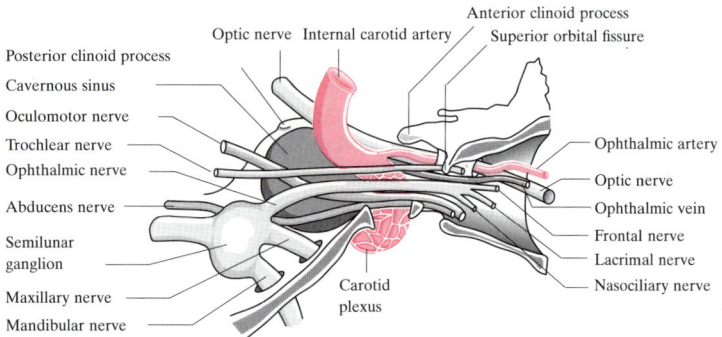

DUANE'S RETRACTION SYNDROME

FORMS OF DUANE'S RETRACTION SYNDROME

[Huber A (1974) Electrophysiology of the retraction syndromes. *Br J Ophthalmol* **58**:293–300]

Type I   Limited or absent abduction
          Restricted adduction
          Narrowing of the lid fissure and retraction of the globe in
              adduction
          Lid fissure widening in attempted abduction
          Face turned to the affected side

Type II   Limited or absent adduction
          Restricted abduction
          Lid fissure narrowing and retraction of the globe in abduction
          Face turned to the unaffected side

Type III Limited or absent abduction and adduction
          Narrowing of the lid fissure and retraction of the globe in
              adduction
          Up- or down-shoot in adduction

ABDUCENS NERVE PALSY VERSUS DUANE'S RETRACTION SYNDROME

	Abducens (VIth) nerve palsy	Duane's syndrome
History	Sudden onset	Congenital
Binocular vision	Diplopia when looking in or towards the field of action of the paretic muscle	Usually no diplopia
Adduction, convergence	Normal	Restricted
Position of the globe	Normal	Retraction in adduction
Lid fissure	Widened in abduction	Narrowed in adduction
Face turn	To the affected side	Not always to the affected side (in type II Duane's syndrome, the patient's face is turned to the unaffected side)

OCULOMOTOR NERVE PALSY: CAUSES

SITES OF LESION AND CAUSES OF OCULOMOTOR NERVE PALSY

Orbit   exophthalmos and various combinations with
             palsies of the IVth and VIth nerves may occur

- posterior orbit tumour (orbital apex syndrome)
- mucocele
- pseudotumour of the orbit
- infection
- trauma

Superior orbital fissure, cavernous sinus

sympathetic plexus lesion and palsies of the III, IV, V and VI nerves may coexist
- carotid cavernous sinus fistula
- tumour (e.g. pituitary adenoma)
- sphenoidal sinusitis
- inflammation (herpes zoster, Tolosa–Hunt syndrome)

Skull base

- increased intracranial pressure, pseudotumour cerebri
- aneurysm (posterior communicating artery, basilar artery, internal carotid artery)
- meningitis (infection: meningococci, Mycobacterium tuberculosis, Treponema pallidum; neoplasm)
- trauma

Mesencephalic brain stem

- ischaemic infarction, haemorrhage
- tumour (e.g. pinealoma)
- inflammation (multiple sclerosis)
- brainstem trauma

Systemic, nonlocalized

- diabetic neuropathy
- infectious (mononucleosis, viral), postvaccination
- migraine

THE PATHWAYS OF THE OCULAR CRANIAL NERVES

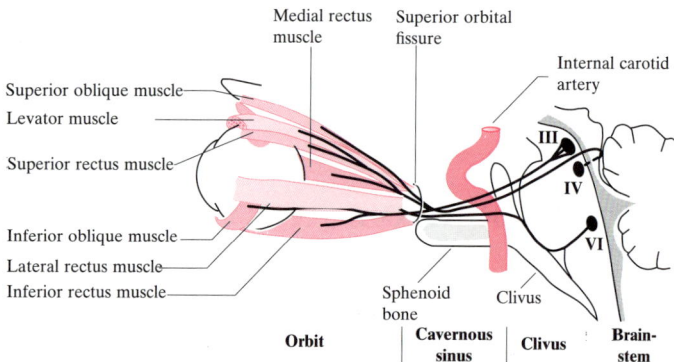

OCULOMOTOR NERVE PALSY: PUPILLARY INVOLVEMENT

Oculomotor nerve palsy	Cause
Affected pupil	Compressive lesion (aneurysm, tumour)
Unaffected pupil	Microangiopathy (diabetes mellitus, hypertension, arteriosclerosis)

Microangiopathies such as hypertension and diabetes mellitus usually involve the vasa nervorum, but spare the pial blood vessels. Due to the superficial location of the pupillomotor fibres in the trunk of the IIIrd nerve, a microangiopathy causing IIIrd nerve palsy will usually spare the pupil. However, lesions such as aneurysms and trauma which compress the pial blood vessels cause IIIrd nerve palsies typically involving the pupil.

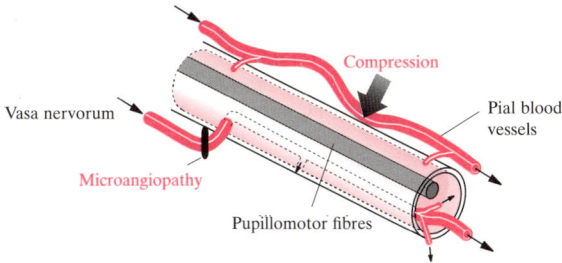

CT/MRI and angiography are urgently indicated in IIIrd nerve palsy with pupillary involvement. In elderly patients with complete oculomotor palsy and no pupillary involvement, invasive investigations may be postponed as long as frequent reviews (at least once weekly) are kept and pupillary involvement or signs of subarachnoid haemorrhage do not occur. If after 6–8 weeks the paresis of the external muscles remains unchanged, the possibility of a compressive lesion without pupillary involvement should be excluded.

In patients under 50 years old and in patients with incomplete IIIrd nerve palsy, CT/MRI and angiography should also be carried out in the presence of an uninvolved pupil, because aneurysms are relatively common in the first group and occult pupillary involvement may occur in the later.

SYMPTOMS OF ANEURYSM-ASSOCIATED SUBARACHNOID HAEMORRHAGE

- Sudden onset of severe headaches
- Nausea, vomiting, drowsiness
- Cranial nerve lesions, especially oculomotor palsy (~20% of all IIIrd nerve palsies are due to a posterior communicating artery aneurysm)

Note: Occasionally, an isolated IIIrd nerve palsy presents as the only symptom of a subarachnoid haemorrhage. Brain CT (even with contrast enhancement) detects aneurysms in only up to 50% of cases. Angiography must therefore be undertaken to exclude an aneurysm. Approximately 90% of terminal subarachnoid harmorrhages are due to an aneurysm.

TROCHLEAR NERVE PALSY: CAUSES

SITES OF LESION AND CAUSES OF TROCHLEAR NERVE PALSY

Orbit
exophthalmos and various combinations with palsies of the IIIrd and VIth nerves may occur
- orbital tumour
- inflammatory orbitopathy
- trauma, ethmoidectomy

Superior orbital fissure, cavernous sinus
sympathetic plexus lesion and palsies of the IIIrd and VIth nerves may coexist
- tumour (nasopharynx)
- carotid cavernous sinus fistula
- intracavernous internal carotid artery aneurysm
- Tolosa–Hunt syndrome, herpes zoster

Skull base
- intracranial pressure
- trauma (involvement of both trochlear nerves possible)
- tumour (pinealoma)
- mastoiditis
- meningitis (infectious, neoplastic)

Mesencephalic brain stem
- inflammation (multiple sclerosis)
- tumour
- ischaemic infarction, haemorrhage
- brain stem trauma

Systemic, nonlocalized
- diabetic neuropathy
- infectious, toxic

BIELSCHOWSKY HEAD TILT TEST

Right trochlear nerve palsy

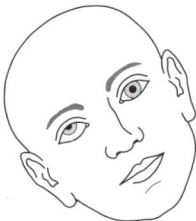

Hyperdeviation of the affected right eye

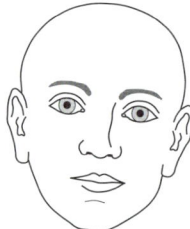

Abnormal head posture (head tilt to the opposite shoulder)

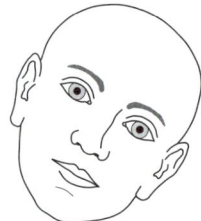

Aligned eyes (no vertical deviation)

Positive Bielschowsky test in **right** IVth nerve palsy: + vertical deviation in forced head tilt to the right.

Positive Bielschowsky test in **left** IVth nerve palsy: − vertical deviation in forced head tilt to the left.

TROCHLEAR NERVE PALSY: DIFFERENTIAL DIAGNOSIS

PARKS THREE-STEP TEST

[Parks MM (1958) Isolated cyclovertical muscle palsy. *Arch Ophthalmol* **60**:1027–1035]

The Parks three-step test is applied in cases of isolated cyclovertical muscle paresis to identify the affected muscle.

1. Which eye shows hyperdeviation?	2. Larger vertical deviation in right or left head tilt?	3. Larger vertical deviation in right or left gaze?	Paretic muscle
Right (+ vertical deviation)	Left tilt	Right gaze	Right inferior rectus
		Left gaze	Left superior rectus
	Right tilt	Right gaze	Left inferior oblique
		Left gaze	Right superior oblique
Left (− vertical deviation)	Left tilt	Right gaze	Left superior oblique
		Left gaze	Right inferior oblique
	Right tilt	Right gaze	Right superior rectus
		Left gaze	Left inferior rectus

UNILATERAL ACQUIRED IVTH NERVE PALSY VERSUS DECOMPENSATED UNILATERAL STRABISMUS SURSOADDUCTORIUS

	Acquired IVth nerve palsy	Decompensated strabismus sursoadductorius
History	Sudden onset	Long-standing head tilt with recent onset of diplopia
Old photographs	No abnormal finding	Head tilt
Abnormal head posture	Acquired since onset	Acquired many years ago, often with the patient being unaware
Largest vertical deviation	Larger vertical deviation in lateral up-gaze than in lateral down-gaze (no inferior oblique over-action)	About the same vertical deviation in lateral up/down-gaze (combination of superior oblique underaction and inferior oblique overaction)
Vertical fusional reserve	Small (in fresh paresis)	Usually large
Excyclotropia	In sursumduction approximately as large as the largest vertical deviation	Concomitant in vertical versions, usually small

Field of single binocular vision	**Acquired IVth nerve palsy** Horizontal dividing line (diplopia in down-gaze)	**Decompensated strabismus sursoadductorius** Vertical dividing line (diplopia in adduction)

Note: The main difference between acquired IVth nerve palsy and decompensated sursoadductorius is that in the first there is no overaction of the ipsilateral inferior oblique. In the latter, there is an overaction of the ipsilateral inferior oblique with a corresponding disorder in the opposite eye. The misleading expression "congenital IVth nerve palsy should not be used anymore.

FACIAL NERVE PALSY

ANATOMICAL RELATIONSHIPS AND FUNCTIONAL COMPONENTS OF THE FACIAL NERVE

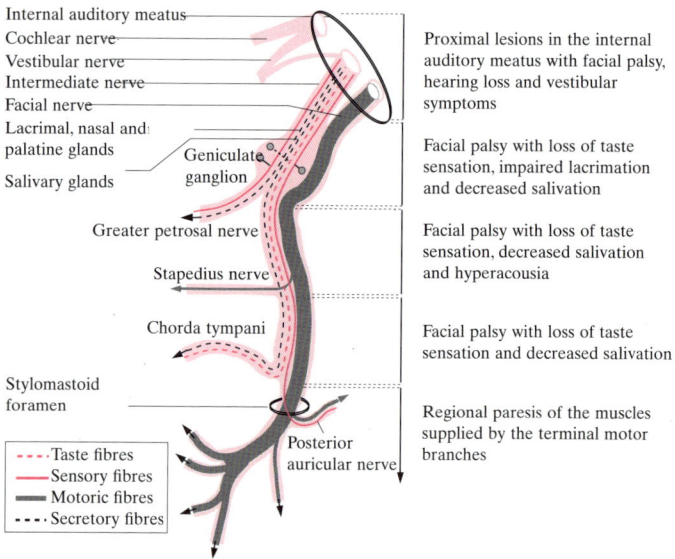

Internal auditory meatus
Cochlear nerve
Vestibular nerve
Intermediate nerve
Facial nerve
Lacrimal, nasal and palatine glands
Salivary glands
Geniculate ganglion
Greater petrosal nerve
Stapedius nerve
Chorda tympani
Stylomastoid foramen
Posterior auricular nerve

- - - Taste fibres
—— Sensory fibres
━━ Motoric fibres
···· Secretory fibres

Proximal lesions in the internal auditory meatus with facial palsy, hearing loss and vestibular symptoms

Facial palsy with loss of taste sensation, impaired lacrimation and decreased salivation

Facial palsy with loss of taste sensation, decreased salivation and hyperacousia

Facial palsy with loss of taste sensation and decreased salivation

Regional paresis of the muscles supplied by the terminal motor branches

Supranuclear VIIth nerve palsy	Weakness of the lower facial muscles; preserved function of the frontalis and orbicularis oculi muscles; unaffected lid closure
Nuclear or peripheral VIIth nerve palsy	Complete facial palsy on the side of the lesion; involvement of both the upper and the lower facial muscles; sagging of the lower lid; widened palpebral fissure; impaired lid closure

MEDICAL TREATMENT FOR BELL'S PALSY (IDIOPATHIC)

[Adour K, Hetzler D (1984) Current medical treatment for facial nerve palsy. *Am J Otol* 5:499–502]

Prednisolone 1 mg/kg in the first 5 days

• Incomplete palsy	Taper off over the next 5 days
• Complete palsy	Continue 1 mg/kg over the next 10 days and taper off over the following 5 days

CRANIAL NERVE SYNDROMES WITH OCULAR INVOLVEMENT

Syndrome	Features
Möbius' syndrome	Bilateral VIth and VIIth nerve palsy with involvement of other cranial nerves; facial weakness (Möbius facies) and difficulty in sucking soon after birth; various oculomotor disorders (horizontal eye movement abnormalities most common); normal pupillary reactions
Benedikt's syndrome	IIIrd nerve palsy with contralateral cerebellar ataxia and tremor; involvement of the red nucleus
Nothnagel's syndrome	IIIrd nerve palsy and ipsilateral cerebellar ataxia; superior cerebellar peduncles lesion
Weber's syndrome	IIIrd nerve palsy with crossed hemiplegia (limbs and face); corticospinal tract lesion in the base of the mid-brain
Raymond–Foville syndrome	Unilateral VIth and VIIth nerve palsy with ipsilateral gaze palsy; ipsilateral Horner's syndrome and deafness may be included; low pontine lesion
Millard–Gubler syndrome	Unilateral VIth and VIIth nerve palsy with contralateral hemiplegia; a more dorsal pontine lesion involving the fascicles of the VI and VIIth nerve and the pyramidal pathways
Wallenberg's syndrome	Ipsilateral Vth, IXth, Xth, XIth nerve palsy, Horner's syndrome and cerebellar ataxia; loss of pain and temperature sensation on the contralateral side of the body; dorsolateral medullary vascular lesion

Syndrome	Features
Gradenigo's syndrome	Otitis media and mastoiditis with secondary petrositis; severe ear pain; VIth nerve palsy with possible involvement of the VIIth, VIIIth and occasionally Vth nerve
Ramsay Hunt' syndrome	Vesicular eruption in the external auditory meatus with ipsilateral VIIth nerve palsy; thought to be caused by herpes zoster of the geniculate ganglion
Superior orbital fissure syndrome	Ophthalmoplegia due to ocular motor nerve compression; e.g. sphenoid ridge meningioma
Cavernous sinus syndrome	Intracavernous lesions lead to involvement of the same nerves as those involved in the superior orbital fissure syndrome; clinical differentiation is therefore difficult and should be supported by orbit and brain imaging
Tolosa–Hunt syndrome	Intense periorbital pain and ipsilateral ophthalmoplegia with separate or combined involvement of the IIIrd, IVth and VIth nerves; granulomatous inflammation of the cavernous sinus
Eaton–Lambert syndrome	Myasthenia-like syndrome secondary to an antiacetylcholine-receptor-antibody-producing neoplasm elsewhere in the body. In contrast to myasthenia gravis, muscle strength increases rather than decreases with voluntary exercise; electromyography shows a recruitment rather than a decrement of motor units in response to repetitive nerve stimulation; ptosis and ophthalmoplegia are often a preterminal sign

SUPRANUCLEAR EYE MOVEMENTS

Malfunction	Lesion
Saccadic system Voluntary and involuntary fast eye movements to objects of interest; quick phases of vestibular and optokinetic nystagmus (OKN)	
Ocular dysmetria (hypermetria, hypometria)	Mainly cerebellar disease
Reduced saccadic velocity	(Pulse generator defect)
Inability to sustain fixation in eccentric gaze, gaze-paretic nystagmus	(Neural integrator defect)

Malfunction	Lesion
Pontine horizontal gaze paresis, internuclear ophthalmoplegia, vertical gaze disturbances	Pontine paramedian reticular formation (PPRF) lesion, medial longitudinal fasciculus (MLF) lesion, rostral interstitial nucleus of the medial longitudinal fasciculus (riMLF) lesion

Smooth pursuit system
Slow eye movements for maintaining fixation on a slow-moving object; slow phases of optokinetic nystagmus

Smooth pursuit asymmetry (right–left OKN asymmetry)	Unilateral cerebral hemisphere lesion (repetitive stimulus movement towards the side of the lesion produces a weaker OKN)
Latent and congenital nystagmus	(Poor temporal monocular smooth pursuit) Often abnormal binocular function

Vestibulo-ocular system
Vestibulo-ocular reflex (VOR); stabilizing the eyes against the sensation of environmental movements

Vestibular nystagmus	Horizontal disorder of VOR
Vertical nystagmus (upbeat nystagmus, downbeat nystagmus)	Medullary lesions and abnormalities of the cervicomedullary junction
Ocular tilt reaction, skew deviation	Posterior fossa disease

Convergence
Disjugate eye movement

Convergence paresis	Usually combined with reduced or absent accommodation (lesion of the Edinger–Westphal nucleus)

SUPRANUCLEAR PATHWAYS

BRAIN-STEM STRUCTURES AND PATHWAYS FOR CONTROL AND COORDINATION OF VOLUNTARY EYE MOVEMENT

Saccadic commands descend from areas of cerebral cortex to decussate at the junction of the mid-brain and pons. They synapse in the anatomically well-defined horizontal gaze centre within the pons called the pontine paramedian reticular formation (PPRF). From the PPRF, the command for horizontal gaze travels to the ipsilateral abducens nucleus and to the lateral rectus muscle; on the other hand, to the contralateral medial longitudinal fasciculus

(MLF) up to the medial rectus subnucleus. The cortical pathways for vertical saccades descend from a less well-defined cerebral area to the rostral interstitial nucleus of the medial longitudinal fasciculus (riMLF). In contrast to the horizontal gaze centre, the vertical gaze centre receives bilateral corticofugal commands.

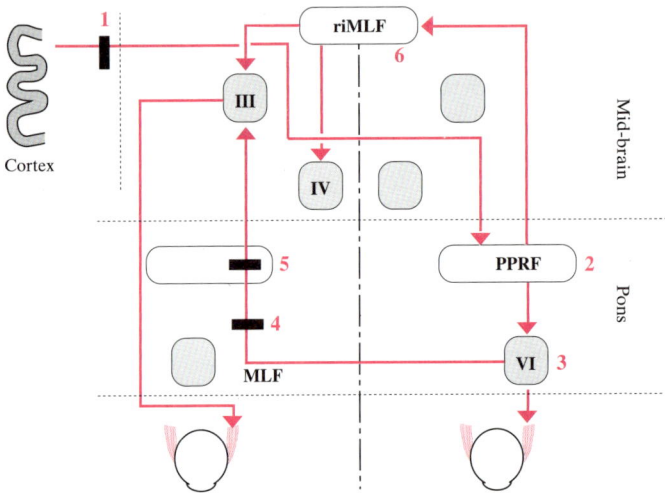

PPRF   Pontine paramedian reticular formation (horizontal gaze centre)
riMLF   Rostral interstitial nucleus of the medial longitudinal fasciculus
        (vertical gaze centre)
MLF   Medial longitudinal fasciculus
III   Oculomotor nucleus
IV   Trochlear nucleus
VI   Abducens nucleus

LOCATION OF LESION

1	Supratentorial lesion	Gaze paresis, preserved smooth pursuit, preserved VOR
2	PPRF lesion	Pontine gaze paresis
3	Abducens nucleus	Combined pontine gaze paresis and abducens paresis
4	MLF lesion	Internuclear ophthalmoplegia
5	Combined lesion of the PPRF and MLF	'One and one-half syndrome' (combined gaze paresis and internuclear ophthalmoplegia)
6	Rostral mid-brain lesion	Vertical gaze disorder and abnormal saccades

SUPRANUCLEAR EYE MOVEMENT DISORDERS

Horizontal gaze paresis with hemiparesis

Patient looks towards the lesion due to inability to produce a horizontal saccade to the contralateral side; the lesion is most commonly a cerebrovascular accident in the cortical distribution of the middle cerebral artery; VOR and smooth pursuit to both sides remain normal; good prognosis

Horizontal pontine gaze paresis

Saccadic horizontal gaze paresis to one side and a hemiparesis on the contralateral side indicate a lesion in the pons; abnormal VOR distinguishes an abducens nucleus lesion from a PPRF lesion; the convergence, which is not controlled by the abducens nucleus, is spared

Dorsal mid-brain syndrome (Parinaud's syndrome)

Typical manifestation of poor or absent up–gaze, light-near dissociation and the pathognomonic convergence–retraction nystagmus; lid retraction (Collier's sign) may also be present; most common cause is a compressive lesion in the pineal region or increased intracranial pressure (e.g. failed shunts)

Internuclear ophthalmoplegia (INO)

Whilst one eye demonstrates loss of adduction, the opposite eye shows an abducting nystagmus; the lesion is ipsilateral to the eye with the adduction deficit; the diagnosis of INO is considered proven if the nonadducting eye responds to a convergence stimulus; mild cases may show only a reduction in the velocity of the adduction saccade.
The lesion is present in the MLF between the VI and contralateral III nucleus; commands from the abducens nucleus cannot travel to the contralateral medial rectus muscle.
Unilateral INO usually affects older patients and is caused by brain-stem infarction; bilateral INO is usually found in younger patients with multiple sclerosis

'One and one-half' syndrome (paralytic pontine exotropia)	Combined horizontal pontine gaze paresis with an INO (palsy of both medial recti and one lateral rectus); lesion affects the MLF, PPRF and abducens nucleus
Ocular tilt reaction	Hypertropia of the contralateral eye, excyclotropia of the ipsilateral eye and a head tilt to the shoulder on the side of the hypotropic eye
Skew deviation	A supranuclear vertical deviation; the disorder can be paroxysmal, transient or permanent; skew deviation is thought to occur as a result of VOR pathway involvement in brain-stem infarctions

DIFFERENTIAL DIAGNOSIS OF SUPRANUCLEAR EYE MOVEMENT DISORDERS

NUCLEAR GAZE DISORDERS VERSUS SUPRANUCLEAR GAZE DISORDERS

- Involvement of all eye movement types (saccades, smooth pursuit, vestibulo-ocular movements, convergence) indicates a nuclear or infranuclear lesion
- An isolated disorder of one eye movement type indicates a supranuclear lesion
- An isolated supranuclear lesion does not cause ocular misalignment. Often, however, supranuclear disorders are combined with nuclear lesions (e.g. nuclear abducens paresis and ipsiversive gaze paresis).

SUSPECTED NUCLEAR EXTRAOCULAR MUSCLE PARESES

Oculomotor	As the nuclei of both sides are adjacent to each other, whereas the nerves are not, bilateral involvement indicates a lesion in the region of the nuclei. A unilateral nuclear oculomotor paresis cannot usually be clinically distinguished from a peripheral oculomotor lesion. A diagnosis of a nuclear oculomotor paresis can usually be made in:

  - bilateral levator paresis without further oculomotor involvement
  - complete oculomotor paresis except for both levators
  - unilateral complete oculomotor paresis with an isolated paresis of the contralateral superior rectus

Trochlear	A nuclear trochlear paresis cannot be clinically distinguished from a peripheral (contralateral) trochlear paresis
Abducens	A nuclear abducens paresis is always associated with a horizontal gaze paresis, because the abducens nucleus

includes two types of neurones: the abducens neurones and the interneurones that decussate to the opposite MLF and to the medial rectus subnucleus.

A coexisting peripheral facial palsy is also suggestive of a lesion in the region of the abducens nucleus.

NYSTAGMUS: CLINICAL EVALUATION

DESCRIBING NYSTAGMUS

Direction of beat (direction of the fast eye movement)	Horizontal (rightbeating, left-beating) Vertical Rotary
Regularity	Regular Irregular
Type	Pendular Jerk Latent
Amplitude	Fine (amplitude $<5°$) Moderate (amplitude $<5–10°$) Coarse (amplitude $>10°$)
Frequency	Low (<1/sec) Moderate ($1–2$/sec) High (>2/sec)
Laterality	Conjugate Dissociated (significant asymmetry)
Cause of nystagmus	Congenital Ocular Vestibular Central

GUIDELINES FOR EVALUATING ABNORMAL OPTOKINETIC NYSTAGMUS (OKN) AND SMOOTH PURSUIT

- Asymmetrical OKN and smooth pursuit without concomitant symptoms (e.g. gaze paresis, nystagmus) indicate a hemispherical lesion. OKN stimulation (e.g. optokinetic drum) shows a weaker OKN towards the side of the lesion.
- Asymmetrical OKN and smooth pursuit in the presence of concomitant symptoms such as marked spontaneous nystagmus, inability to hold the eyes in eccentric gaze, or paralysis suggest a brain stem lesion or a cerebellar lesion.
- A symmetrical disoder of OKN and smooth pursuit with gaze-evoked nystagmus is most commonly drug-induced (e.g. sedatives, tranquilizers).

- Disorder of OKN and smooth pursuit with a nystagmus that increases with fixation indicate congenital nystagmus.

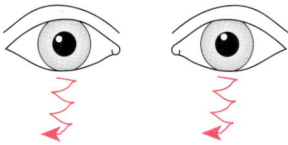

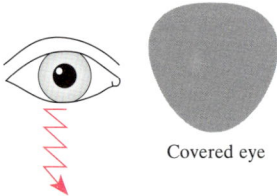

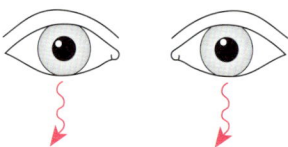

SYNOPSIS OF NYSTAGMUS TYPES

Nystagmus types

Physiological nystagmus	Occurs in extreme lateral gaze and demonstrates a horizontal nystagmus with small amplitude and jerk component to the side of gaze.
Rebound nystagmus	A gaze-evoked nystagmus that decreases its amplitude when an eccentric gaze is sustained and then rebounds, reversing its direction (associated with cerebellar dysfunction).
Square wave jerks	Fixation instability in systemic degenerations of the basal ganglia and cerebellum. May occur physiologically in a tired or exhausted person.
Congenital nystagmus	Begins at birth or during the first three months of life; horizontal pendular nystagmus in primary position; jerk nystagmus on lateral gaze; decreases with convergence; increases with fixation; abnormal head posture due to a null point outside the primary position.
Latent nystagmus	A jerk nystagmus that occurs or increases its intensity when binocular vision is disrupted (one eye covered). The fast component is towards the fixing eye. Often associated with congenital esotropia.
Deprivation nystagmus	Horizontal pendular nystagmus in congenital or acquired (2–6 years old) bilateral visual loss.
Acquired pendular nystagmus in neurological diseases	Horizontal, often asymmetric, pendular nystagmus. OKN and saccades usually uninvolved. Most commonly associated with multiple sclerosis.

Covered eye

Superior oblique myokymia   Monocular episodic oscillation which can often be brought out in down-gaze. Treatment with carbamazepine may help. Otherwise, surgical weakening of the ipsilateral superior oblique muscle is indicated.

Vestibular nystagmus   Central or peripheral vestibular nystagmus. Usually with rotary movements. Most commonly with vertigo, tinnitus and hearing loss. In central vestibular nystagmus, fixation does not inhibit the nystagmus. In peripheral vestibular nystagmus, the slow component of the nystagmus is towards the lesion.

Gaze-evoked nystagmus   No nystagmus in primary position. Jerk nystagmus occurs in eccentric gaze position. Fast component in the direction of gaze. In the absence of further symptoms, a gaze-evoked nystagmus is nonspecific for anatomical location.

Gaze-paretic nystagmus   Occurs when a paretic muscle is unable to hold the eye in eccentric gaze. Often not to be differentiated from gaze-evoked nystagmus.

Spasmus nutans   High-frequency oscillations. Usually bilateral but asymmetrical. Concomitant head nodding and abnormal head postures often present. Begins in the first year of life and usually resolves after one or two years. Intracranial tumours may coexist. Computed imaging for exclusion of tumour is therefore indicated.

See-saw nystagmus

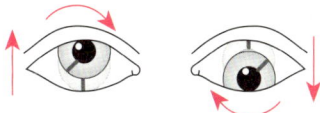

A dissociation nystagmus in which one eye moves up and incyclorotates as the other eye moves down and excyclorotates. In children often associated with parasellar tumours.

Dissociated nystagmus

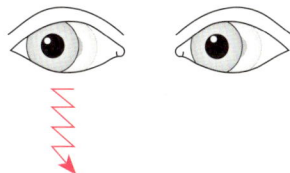

A horizontal gaze-paretic nystagmus that in internuclear ophthalmoplegia occurs only in the abducting eye, but in both eyes in multiple sclerosis.

Convergence–retraction nystagmus

Occurs spontaneously or in attempted upgaze (best tested with downgoing optokinetic drum). Associated with the dorsal mid-brain symdrome (Parinaud's syndrome, pinealoma).

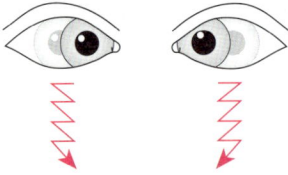

Downbeat nystagmus

Vertical nystagmus with downbeating fast component. Increases in lateral gaze. Not inhibited in fixation. Most commonly associated with spinocerebellar degenerations.

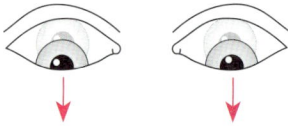

Upbeat nystagmus

Vertical nystagmus with upbeating fast component. Not inhibited in fixation. The amplitude of the nystagmus depends on the anatomical location of the lesion. When an upbeat nystagmus is not present in the primary position, it is a nonspecific gaze-evoked nystagmus.

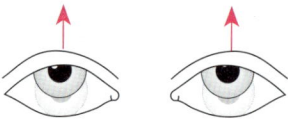

Periodic alternating nystagmus

Periodic horizontal jerk nystagmus which alternates from one direction to the other. The amplitude of the nystagmus gradually increases and decreases in each direction. Most commonly associated with pontomedullar lesions.

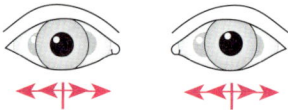

Opsoclonus

Constant or intermittent, chaotic fast eye movements in random directions. Most commonly associated with viral encephalitis. Coexisting ataxia or limb myoclonus may indicate a cerebellar lesion.

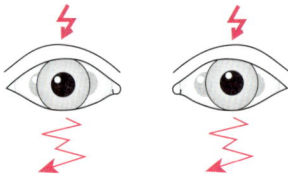

Ocular bobbing

Fast down movement of the eyes with a slow return movement to primary position. Usually occurs in the comatose patient with pontal lesion and loss of horizontal eye movements.

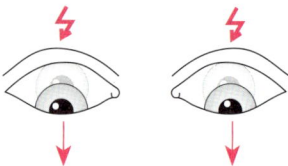

Ocular myoclonus   Spontaneous vertical pendular nystagmus. It can be associated with myocloni of the palate (oculopalatal myoclonus) and is then indicative of a brain-stem lesion.

HEADACHE

DIAGNOSTIC CRITERIA OF OPHTHALMIC-RELATED HEADACHE SYNDROMES

[Headache Classification Committee of the International Headache Society (1988) Classification and diagnostic criteria for headache disorders, cranial neuralgia and facial pain. *Cephalgia* **8 (Suppl 7)**: 1–93]

Migraine without aura (common migraine)
A. A total of at least five attacks
B. Duration of attack 4–72 hours
C. At least two of the following criteria are present: unilateral manifestation, pulsating pain, moderate to severe intensity, increased intensity with physical strain
D. At least one of the following criteria is present during the painful stage: nausea and vomiting, photosensitivity, sensitivity to noise

Migraine with aura (classic migraine)
A. A total of at least two attacks
B. One or more of the following aura symptoms: homonymous visual defects, unilateral paraesthesia and/or sensory deficit, unilateral paresis, speech disorder
C. No aura symptom persists longer than 60 minutes. The aura precedes the pain with an interval of less than 60 minutes, but also can occur during or after the painful stage

Ophthalmoplegic migraine
A. At least two attacks
B. Headache plus paresis of one or several cranial nerves (III, IV, VI)
C. Other causes to be excluded (sella, cavernous sinus, superior orbital fissure). Often difficult to differentiate from Tolosa–Hunt syndrome

Episodic tension-type headache
A. A total of at least 10 attacks, but <180 headache days per year or <15 per month
B. Duration of painful stage between 30 minutes and 7 days
C. At least two of the following criteria are present: bilateral manifestation, pressing (not pulsating) pain, mild to moderate intensity, unchanged intensity with physical strain
D. No aura

Cluster headache
A. A total of at least five attacks
B. Severe unilateral orbital, supraorbital or temporal pain. Duration of an untreated attack 15–180 minutes

C. At least one of the following criteria is present: conjunctival injection, lacrimation, nasal congestion, rhinorrhoea, severe sweating of the forehead and face, Horner's syndrome, lid oedema
D. Frequency of attacks is between one attack every other day and eight attacks per day

Giant cell arteritis
A. One or more of the following criteria: swollen and tender superficial artery in the region of the scalp or the head (usually the superficial temporal artery), elevated erythrocyle sedimentation rate, symptomatic relief 48 hours after commencement of systemic corticosteroid therapy
B. Confirmation of diagnosis with biopsy of the superficial temporal artery

Benign intracranial hypertension (pseudotumour cerebri)
A. The following criteria are obligatory:
   Elevated intracranial pressure >200 mm H_2O
   No neurological abnormalities other than papilloedema or abducens paresis
   CT or MRI show no mass and normal or small ventricles
   Normal cerebrospinal fluid
   No cavernous sinus thrombosis
B. Intensity and frequency of the headaches corresponds to the intracranial pressure

Tolosa–Hunt syndrome
A. One or more episodes of unilateral orbital pain. Duration of an untreated attack ~8 weeks
B. Paresis of one or several cranial nerves (III, IV, VI) within the first two weeks
C. Symptomatic relief 72 hours after commencement of systemic corticosteroid therapy

Idiopathic trigeminal neuralgia
A. Paroxysmal facial or forehead pain attacks. Duration of the painful stage 2 sec–2 min
B. The pain includes at least four of the following criteria:
   Distribution along one or several branches of the trigeminal nerve
   Sudden, sharp, superficial, stabbing or burning pain
   Severe intensity of pain
   Stimulation of the affected trigeminal-innervated area by touch or with certain daily activities such as drinking, brushing the teeth etc.
   No symptoms between attacks
C. No neurological deficit
D. The attacks of a certain patient follow the same pattern

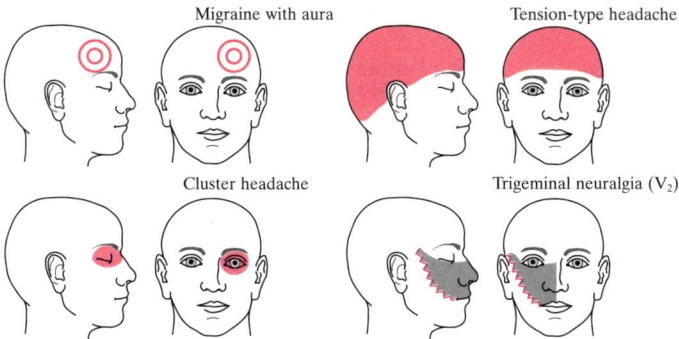

Migraine with aura

Tension-type headache

Cluster headache

Trigeminal neuralgia (V_2)

ABERRANT INNERVATION

ABERRANT INNERVATIONS WITH OCULAR INVOLVEMENT

Voluntary movement	Involuntary comovement	Features
Oculomotor nerve (medial rectus)	Oculomotor nerve (levator palpebrae)	Upper lid retraction in adduction, aberrant regeneration after traumatic oculomotor paresis
Oculomotor nerve (medial rectus)	Oculomotor nerve (inferior rectus)	Depression in adduction, retraction
Oculomotor nerve (medial rectus)	Oculomotor nerve (superior rectus)	Elevation in adduction, retraction
Oculomotor nerve (medial rectus, vertical motors)	Oculomotor nerve (pupillomotor fibres, ciliary ganglion)	Miosis in adduction and attempted supraduction
Oculomotor nerve (medial rectus)	Abducens nerve	Duane's syndrome
Trigeminal nerve (lateral pterygoid muscle)	Oculomotor nerve (levator palpebrae)	Marcus Gunn's 'jaw-winking' syndrome, mandibulopalpebral synkinesis
Trigeminal nerve (chewing)	Facial nerve (orbicularis oculi)	Martin–Amat syndrome, (increased) ptosis whilst chewing
Trigeminal nerve	Trochlear nerve	Eye movements whilst swallowing
Trigeminal nerve	Abducens nerve	Abduction when putting teeth together

Voluntary movement	Involuntary comovement	Features
Abducens nerve	Oculomotor nerve (levator palpebrae)	Upper lid elevation in abduction
Abducens nerve	Facial nerve (obicularis oculi)	Upper lid depression in abduction
Facial nerve (platysma)	Oculomotor nerve	Reduced ptosis when mouth is turned down
Facial nerve	Trigeminal nerve	Opening of the mouth when attempting to overcome orbicularis spasm
Facial nerve (parotid gland)	Facial nerve (lacrimal gland)	Crocodile tears

Chapter 12

ORBIT

THE ORBITAL CAVITY

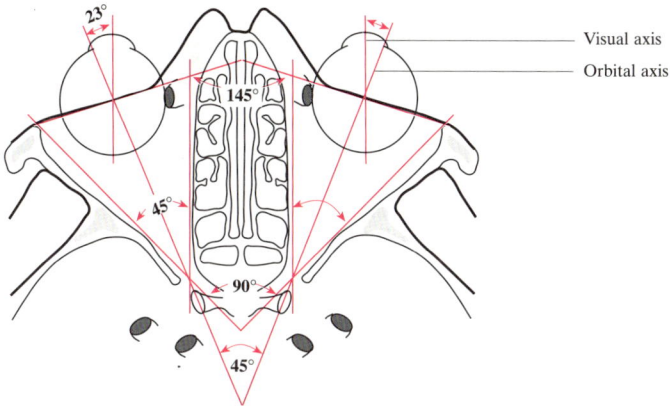

The medial wall is situated anteroposteriorly in the sagittal plane; the lateral wall runs at an angle of approximately 45°. The average angle between the orbital axis and the visual axis is approximately 23°.

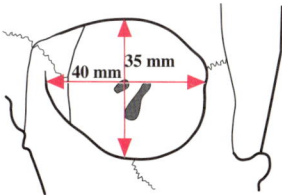

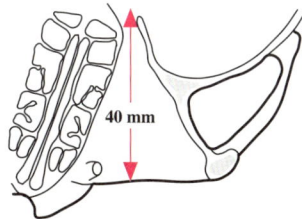

ANATOMY OF THE ORBIT

THE BONY STRUCTURES OF THE ORBIT

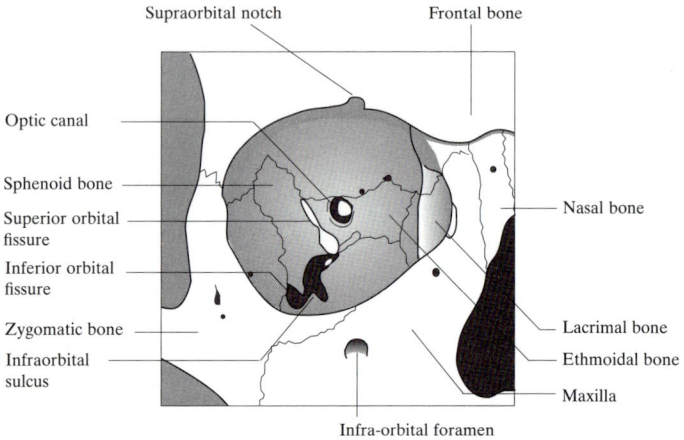

APEX OF THE ORBITAL CAVITY

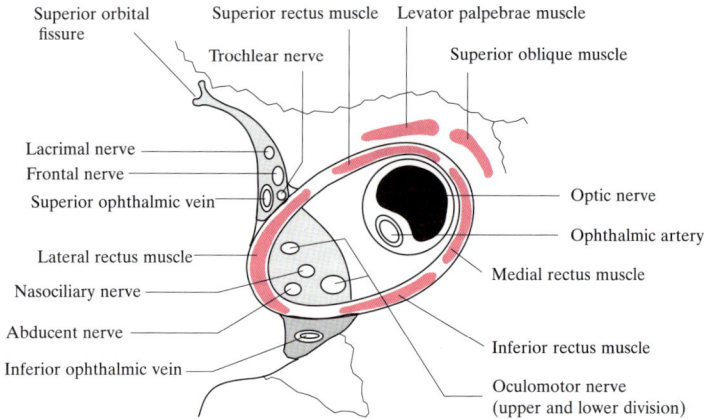

ORDER OF NERVES IN THE SUPERIOR ORBITAL FISSURE

Top to bottom:

Outside the tendinous ring:
   Lacrimal nerve (V_1)
   Frontal nerve (V_1)
   Trochlear nerve
Within the tendinous ring:
   Oculomotor nerve (upper division)
   Nasociliary nerve (V_1)
   Abducent nerve
   Oculomotor nerve (lower division)

SURFACE ANATOMY OF THE ORBIT

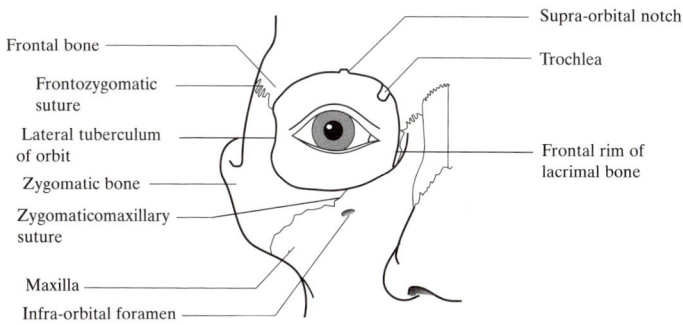

Frontal bone
Frontozygomatic suture
Lateral tuberculum of orbit
Zygomatic bone
Zygomaticomaxillary suture
Maxilla
Infra-orbital foramen

Supra-orbital notch
Trochlea
Frontal rim of lacrimal bone

OPENINGS INTO THE ORBITAL CAVITY AND THE STRUCTURES THAT RUN THROUGH THEM

Opening	Contents
Optic canal	Optic nerve, ophthalmic artery
Superior orbital fissure	Oculomotor nerve (III), trochlear nerve (IV), abducent nerve (VI), ophthalmic nerve (V_1), ophthalmic vein, sympathetic fibres
Inferior orbital fissure	Inferior ophthalmic vein
Foramen rotundum	Maxillary nerve (V_2)
Supraorbital notch	Supraorbital nerve, supraorbital vessels
Infraorbital foramen	Infraorbital nerve (V_2), infraorbital artery

RELATIONSHIPS OF THE SINUSES TO THE ORBIT

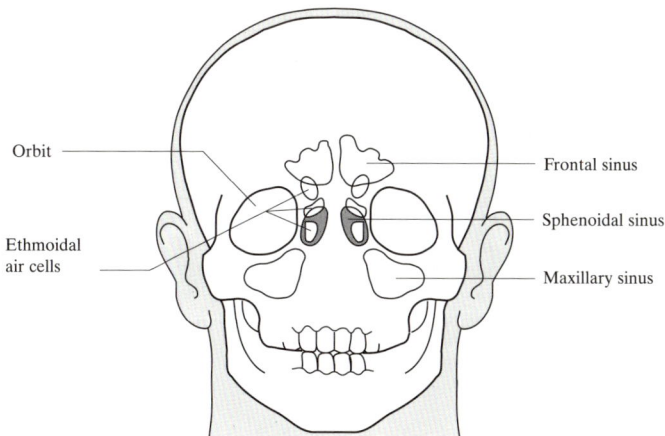

Orbit
Ethmoidal air cells

Frontal sinus
Sphenoidal sinus
Maxillary sinus

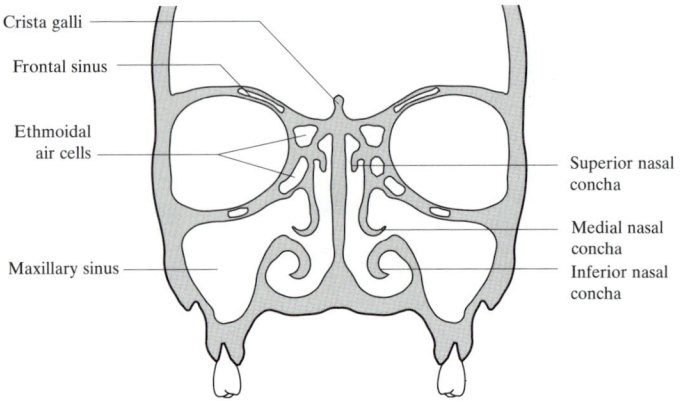

Crista galli
Frontal sinus
Ethmoidal air cells
Maxillary sinus

Superior nasal concha
Medial nasal concha
Inferior nasal concha

THE ORBITAL BLOOD VESSELS

ARTERIES WITHIN THE ORBITAL CAVITY

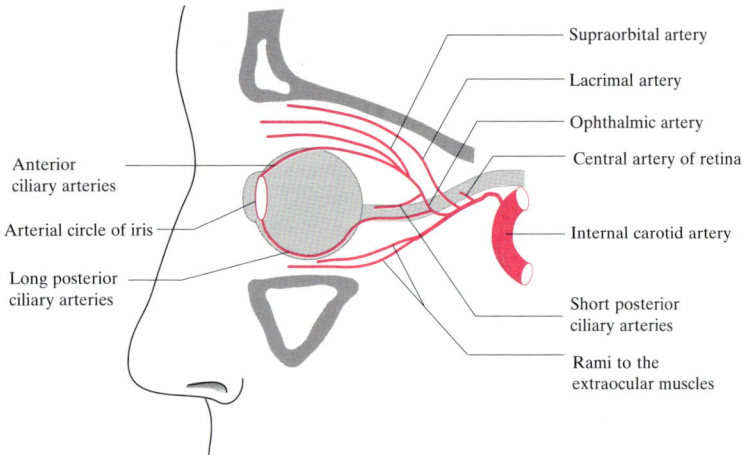

Anterior ciliary arteries
Arterial circle of iris
Long posterior ciliary arteries

Supraorbital artery
Lacrimal artery
Ophthalmic artery
Central artery of retina
Internal carotid artery
Short posterior ciliary arteries
Rami to the extraocular muscles

VEINS WITHIN THE ORBITAL CAVITY

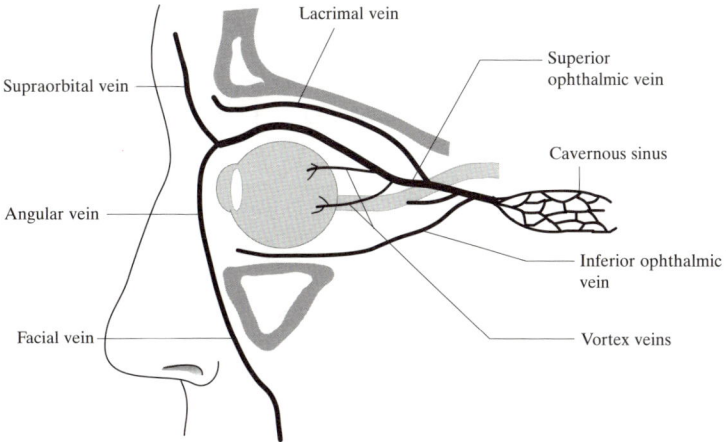

ORBITAL RADIOGRAPH –
OCCIPITOFRONTAL OBLIQUE VIEW

OCCIPITOFRONTAL OBLIQUE VIEW

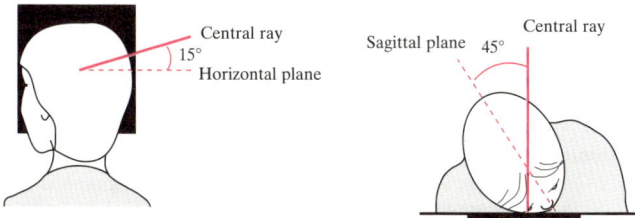

Patient's position:	Turn the head 45° away from the side under examination. The outer orbital rim, apex of the nose and cheek are in contact with the X-ray table. The orbit is placed in the centre of the film. The central ray is tilted 10–15° craniocaudally.
Evaluation:	• Orbital apex
	• Optic canal (the central ray is orthograde to the optic canal of the orbit under examination)
	• Angled view of the posterior ethmoidal air cells
	• Clinoid process of the lesser sphenoidal wing
	• Radiographs of both sides should be taken (the diameter of the optic canal measures 3.5–5.5 mm: a difference of more than 1 mm between the diameters of the right and left optic canals is pathological)

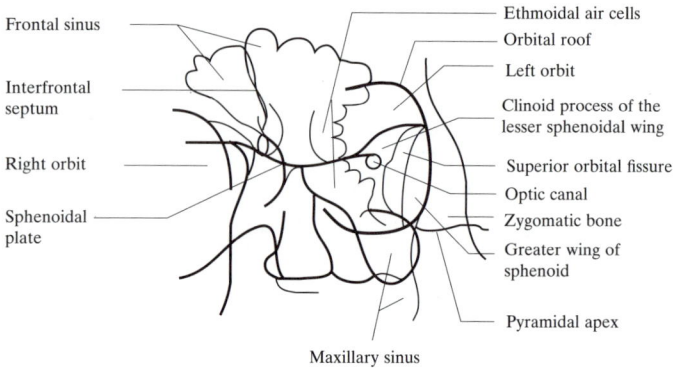

Frontal sinus

Interfrontal septum

Right orbit

Sphenoidal plate

Ethmoidal air cells

Orbital roof

Left orbit

Clinoid process of the lesser sphenoidal wing

Superior orbital fissure

Optic canal

Zygomatic bone

Greater wing of sphenoid

Pyramidal apex

Maxillary sinus

ORBITAL RADIOGRAPH – OCCIPITOMENTAL VIEW (WATERS' VIEW)

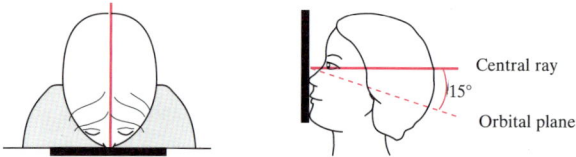

Central ray

15°

Orbital plane

Patient's position: Place the nose and chin in contact with the midline of the X-ray table. The median sagittal plane is at right angles to the film. the central ray is at 15° to the orbital plane (the orbital plane travels along the upper margin of the external acoustic meatus and the lowest point of the inferior orbital rim).

Evaluation:
- Good view of the lower orbital rim enables detection of orbital floor fractures (although CT is indicated for exclusion of the same)
- Also good view of the frontal sinuses, ethmoidal air cells and to a lesser degree the maxillary sinuses
- A Comberg shell is used to demonstrate the location of a suspected intraorbital foreign body (although nowadays CT is the preferred method for imaging intra-orbital foreign bodies, giving precise location without the discomfort of an epicorneal shell. MRI provides similar advantages, but is contraindicated for metallic foreign bodies)

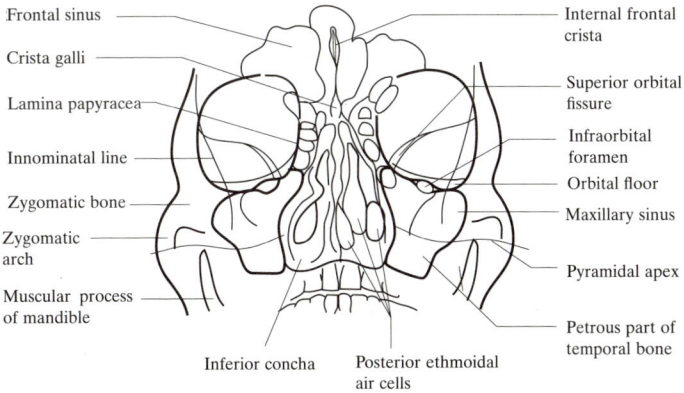

ORBITAL DISEASE – EXAMINATION

HERTEL EXOPHTHALMOMETER

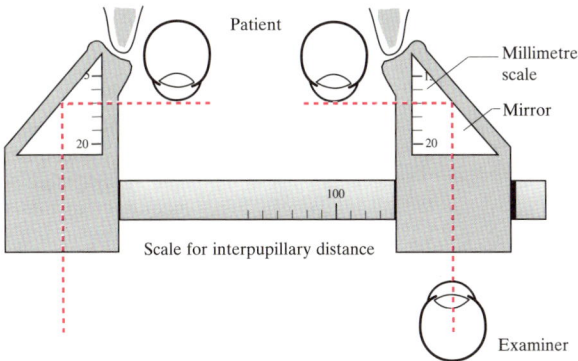

NORMAL MEASUREMENTS

The upper normal limit of exophthalmometry for the Hertel instrument is usually 18 mm; 19 mm for the Krahn instrument.

A previously measured 15 mm which now measures 18 mm must also be considered as evidence for exophthalmos.

A difference of more than 2 mm between the two eyes is considered abnormal.

In addition to measurement with the exophthalmometer, the presence of an exophthalmos should be estimated as follows: the examiner stands behind the sitting patient, lifts both upper lids and looks for a difference between the curvature of the lower lid margins.

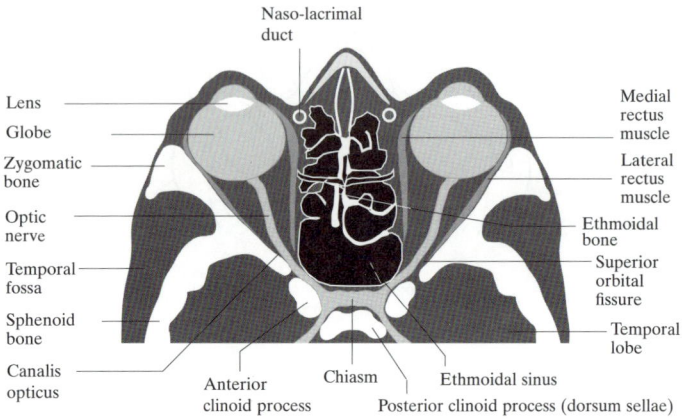

DIFFERENTIAL DIAGNOSIS OF EXOPHTHALMOS

TUMOURS

Meningioma

Medial aspect of sphenoid	Periorbital pain and mid-forehead headaches; compression of the I, III, V_1 and other cranial nerves
Lateral aspect of sphenoid	Full temporalis fossa secondary to hyperostosis; temporal headache; proptosis and optic nerve compression
Optic nerve sheath	Can occur at any age but most commonly seen in middleaged women; intraconal, usually unilateral, slowgrowing, benign tumour; optociliary shunt vessels are typical but they may also occur in optic nerve glioma; calcifications on CT
Lymphoma	Usually of non-Hodgkin type; more common in elderly people; often without signs of systemic neoplasm; palpable lesions may occur due to anterior orbital involvement
Leukaemic infiltrates	Often bilateral; not infrequently with concomitant choroidal or retinal changes
Neurofibromatosis	Ocular features include, neuroma, meningioma, optic nerve glioma, buphthalmos, mucocele (in congenital sphenoid bone defect)

Lymphangioma	Slowly progressive proptosis in childhood; intermittent haemorrhages which may lead to sudden proptosis with formation of large dark masses (chocolate cysts)
Cavernous haemangioma	Most common orbital tumour in adults; usually intra-conal, slowly growing tumour; in contrast to optic nerve tumours, CT typically shows sparing of the orbital apex; surgical excision usually possible
Capillary haemangioma	Common; usually located in the anterior orbit and apparent at birth; increase in size when the baby cries
Rhabdomyosarcoma	Most common primary orbital tumour in childhood (average age seven years), rapidly-progressive, highly malignant
Optic nerve glioma (juvenile pilocytic astrocytoma)	Most commonly seen in young children; usually unilateral; slowly progressive visual loss and proptosis; in late stages the proptosis may cause inferotemporal displacement of the eye; extension into the arachnoid space is characteristic when associated with neurofibromatosis
Neuroblastoma	Embryonal malignant tumour; orbital metastases are common; presentation usually before three years of age
Metastases	Orbital metastases are less common than intra-ocular metastases; prognosis for survival is usually poor; in female adults the most common sites for the primary tumour are the breast and lung, in men the prostate and lung; in children, the most common metastases include neuroblastoma, leukaemia and Ewing's sarcoma

INFLAMMATIONS

Graves' ophthalmopathy	Usually bilateral but may be asymmetric; approximately 5% of patients are euthyroid; CT/MRI shows enlargement of the involved muscles with sparing of the tendons; most commonly affected muscle is the inferior rectus. 'Orbital myositis' usually indicates idiopathic inflammation of muscle
Orbital pseudotumour	Inflammatory process of unknown origin; bilateral involvement indicates a systemic disease (e.g. lymphoma, Wegener's granulomatosis, tuberculosis, sarcoidosis)

Tolosa–Hunt syndrome	Granulomatous inflammation of the cavernous sinus; intense periorbital pain; separate or combined paresis of the III, IV and VI nerves; improvement with corticosteroid therapy does not prove the diagnosis – however, no improvement suggests a different cause.
Acute orbital myositis	Redness and pain over the affected muscle (one or several muscles may be involved); CT shows enlargement of the involved muscles including the tendons
Orbital phlegmon	Most common after trauma
Orbital mucormycosis	Most commonly affects immunosuppressed patients; treatment includes amphotericin B and surgical excision

VASCULAR ABNORMALITIES

Orbital varices	Intermittent exophthalmos which typically increases in size with jugular vein compression or Valsalva manoeuvre; ultrasound and CT often show phleboliths
Arteriovenous fistula	
High-flow fistula	Usually a defect in the wall of the intracavernous portion of the internal carotid artery often related to head trauma; eyelid swelling, chemosis, pulsating proptosis, audible bruit, ophthalmoplegia
Low-flow fistula	Usually a spontaneous indirect connection (dural arterial vessels) between the cavernous sinus and the internal carotid artery; engorged episcleral vessels, mild proptosis, mild ocular motor nerve involvement; diagnosis is made with angiography
Cavernous sinus thrombosis	Acute presentation; headaches, elevated body temperature, vomiting, ophthalmoplegia; usually bilateral proptosis
Orbital haematoma	Post traumatic

OTHER CAUSES FOR PROPTOSIS

Mucocele	Cystic lesions following chronic sinusitis, most commonly frontal and ethmoidal sinuses; slowly progressive, painless proptosis with downward or lateral displacement of the globe
Craniofacial dysplasia	
Craniofacial dysostosis (Crouzon's syndrome)	Premature synotosis of the coronal and sagittal sutures; hypertelorism; small orbits; increased intraocular pressure possible (optic atrophy)
Mandibulofacial dysplasia (Franceschetti–Zwahlen syndrome)	Antimongoloid eyelid position; microgenia; inferior displacement of the ear

Oculoauricular dysplasia (Goldenhar's syndrome)	Antimongoloid eyelid position; malformations of the external ear and deafness; epibulbar lipodermoids adjacent to the limbus
Hypertelorism (Greig's syndrome)	Arrested embryonal medial transposition of the orbits; laterofixation of the orbits
Osteopathies	Paget's disease; Hurler's multiplex dysostosis (gargoylism); Albers–Schönberg ('marble bones' disease).
Meningocele, encephalocele	Congenital dehiscences of the skull which may cause herniation of intracranial content into the orbit; congenital sphenoid bone defects in neurofibromatosis may produce pulsating proptosis
Histiocytosis X (Langerhans-cell histiocytosis)	Three rare disorders (Hand–Schüller–Christian disease, Letterer–Siwe syndrome, eosinophilic granuloma) whilst differing in the extent of organ involvement and prognosis, are unified by the presence of histiocyte-like cells in the lesions; the first two conditions classically affect young children; eosinophilic granuloma occurs in children and young adults; orbital involvement can lead to the triad of bony lesions, diabetes insipidus and exophthalmos
Parasites	Cysticercosis (*Taenia solium*), orbital *Echinococcus*, ophthalmomyiasis (caused by maggots of certain fly species).

CHARACTERISTIC LOCATION OF COMMON ORBITAL DISEASES

Intraconal	Extraconal	Muscular
Cavernous haemangioma	Dermoid	Graves' ophthalmopathy
Optic nerve glioma	Sphenoid meningioma	Rhabdomyosarcoma
Optic nerve sheath meningioma	Lacrimal gland tumour	

Neurofibromatosis, lymphangioma and pseudotumours occur in all three locations.

GRAVES' OPHTHALMOPATHY

- Found in up to two-thirds of patients with autoimmune hyperthyroidism.
- May also be found in euthyroid patients with normal antibody levels.

Clinical signs of Graves' ophthalmopathy

Dalrymple's sign	Lid retraction
von Graefe's sign	Upper lid lag in down-gaze
Stellwag's sign	Reduced frequency of blink
Möbius' sign	Poor convergence

Werner's classification of ocular signs of Graves' ophthalmopathy (American Thyroid Association)

[Werner SC (1969) Classification of the eye changes in Graves' disease. *J Clin Endocrinol Metab* **29**: 982–984]

I   Lid retraction (Müller's muscle)
II   Involvement of the lids and conjunctiva (chemosis)
III   Proptosis
IV   Extraocular muscle thickening, motility disorders, increased intraocular
      pressure in upgaze compared with primary position
V   Corneal involvement (lagophthalmos)
VI   Optic nerve compression

Note: All the above manifestations can occur in any order.

Management

Conservative	Dark glasses, lubricants, raised head position at night
Corticosteroids	Prednisolone 60–100 mg daily to be gradually decreased over 4 weeks, then maintenance dosage of 5–10 mg daily for at least 3–4 months
Radiation therapy	6–10 Gy in 1–2 Gy daily sessions; may be combined with highdose systemic steroid therapy
Surgical decompression	Various techniques exist; sufficient orbital apex decompression should be achieved
Strabismus surgery	Inferior rectus muscle is most commonly involved (fibrosis of the muscle causes restricted supraduction)

NEUROFIBROMATOSIS/NON-HODGKIN LYMPHOMA

DIAGNOSTIC CRITERIA OF NEUROFIBROMATOSIS

[National Institute of Health Consensus Development Conference (1988) Neurofibromatosis: conference statement. *Arch Neurol* **45**: 575–578]

Neurofibromatosis type I

The diagnosis is established when two or more of the following symptoms are present:

- six or more café-au-lait spots (minimum diameter 1.5 cm, 0.5 cm in pre-puberty years)
- two or more neurofibromas or a plexiform neurofibroma
- axillary freckling
- optic nerve glioma
- two or more iris hamartomas
- sphenoid bone defects causing pulsating proptosis

Neurofibromatosis type II (less common than type I)

The diagnosis is based on the following criterion:

• Bilateral acoustic neuroma

If the patient has a close relative with neurofibromatosis type II, the diagnosis can be made on two of the following criteria:

• neurofibroma
• meningioma
• glioma
• schwannoma
• juvenile posterior subcapsular cataract

CLASSIFICATION OF NON-HODGKIN LYMPHOMA (1977)

[National Cancer Institute (1982) Sponsored study of classifications of non-Hodgkin's lymphomas. Summary and description of working formulation for clinical usage. *Cancer* **49**: 2112]

Low grade

a. Small lymphocytic
b. Follicular, predominantly small cleaved cell
c. Follicular, mixed small cleaved and large cell

Intermediate grade

d. Follicular, predominantly large cell
e. Diffuse, small cleaved cell
f. Diffuse, mixed small and large cell
g. Diffuse, large cell

High grade

h. Large cell, immunoblastic
i. Lymphoblastic
j. Small non-cleaved cell

Chapter 13

PUPIL

PUPILLARY REACTIONS: APPLIED NEUROANATOMY

LIGHT REFLEX AND ACCOMMODATION

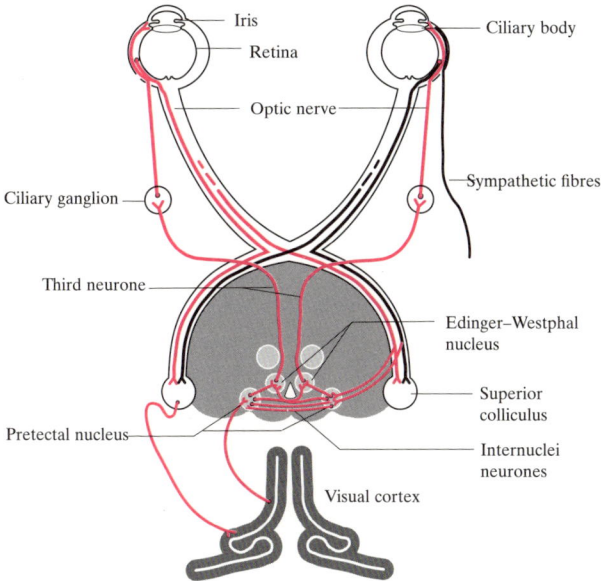

Neuroconnections of the light reflex (right) and accommodation (left)

APPLIED PHARMACOLOGY

Miosis		Mydriasis	
Parasympathomimetic drugs		Parasympatholytic drugs	
Direct	*Indirect*	Atropine	
Acetylcholine	Physostigmine	Scopolamine	
Pilocarpine	(Eserine)	Homatropine	
Aceclidine	Carbachol	Cyclopentolate	
Carbachol		Tropicamide	
Sympatholytic drugs		Sympathomimetic drugs	
Guanethidine		*Direct*	*Indirect*
Dapiprazole		Adrenaline	Cocaine
		Phenylephrine	Dopamine
		Dipivefrine	Pholedrine
		Naphazoline	Tyramine
		Xylometazoline	
		Clonidine	

PUPILLARY REACTIONS: EXAMINATION

WORK-UP AND INTERPRETATION OF PUPILLARY DYSFUNCTION

Work-up

First check for anisocoria and pupillary reaction to light. Establish whether there is a unilateral or bilateral pupillary dysfunction. Always check the pupillary size in a bright, evenly lit room and in relative darkness.

Next use the swinging flashlight test to check for an afferent pupillary defect. This is best done in a darkened room with the patient looking to the far end of the room to avoid a near reflex.

The near reflex consists of accommodation, convergence of the visual axes and constriction of the pupils. It is carried out on a target with the same luminescence as the far target.

Interpretation

If there is no anisocoria in either darkness or light and if the pupillary reactions to light are normal, then there is no efferent or supranuclear pupillary dysfunction. Increased anisocoria in darkness indicates dilation insufficiency, whereas worsening in brighter light indicates constriction insufficiency.

A relative afferent pupillary defect (Marcus Gunn pupil) typically indicates a unilateral optic nerve lesion, although it can also be caused by advanced retinal lesions.

There is no clinical condition with an isolated lesion of the pupils near constriction. It is always combined with lesions of accomodation, convergence or pupillary reaction to light. Light–near dissociation is present if the light reflex is absent or abnormal but the near response is intact.

OTHER NORMAL PUPILLARY REFLEXES

Physiological pupillary unrest

The normal pupillary movement goes on constantly, even when the stimulation of the pupil does not vary. It is strongly light-dependent.

Ciliospinal skin reflex

Pinching the skin at the neck dilates the pupils via the pain fibres of the descending branch of the fifth cranial nerve.

Tournay phenomenon

This term refers to dilation of the pupil in the abducting eye on sustained lateral gaze. The reaction does not occur immediately but after a few seconds of retained gaze and is probably caused by asymmetric accommodative convergence in side gaze, as may be seen in exophoric patients who compensate their exophoria with accommodative convergence. The phenomenon is always benign and may also be seen in normal subjects.

SYNOPSIS OF PUPILLARY DISORDERS

Diagnosis	Cause	Pupil	Comment
Amaurotic pupil	Unilateral blindness	No anisocoria; convergence present; positive swinging flashlight test with present efferent reaction	Absolute afferent pupillary defect, i.e. optic nerve atrophy
Oculomotor palsy with pupillary involvement	Suspected IIIrd nerve compression	Increased anisocoria in bright light (constriction insufficiency); absent direct reaction to light and absent near response	Always exclude IIIrd nerve compression urgently (compressive lesion of the third nerve due to posterior communicating aneurysm is usually associated with severe pain)
Parinaud's syndrome	Dorsal mid-brain lesion	Poor light reaction, better near reaction (light–near dissociation)	Most common causes are pinealomas and hydrocephalus (look for poor or absent upgaze and convergence–retraction nystagmus)
Drug-induced cycloplegia	Cycloplegic drugs; contact with sap from certain plants and flowers (many of the night-blooming flowers contain scopolamine)	Mydriasis; insufficient pupillary constriction to 1% pilocarpine	In third-nerve palsy, the motor end-plates are intact and the pupil responds appropriately to application of 1% pilocarpine
Anxiety-induced mydriasis	Sympathetic hyperactivity	Bilateral large pupils with decreased reaction to light and near stimulus	After ease of anxiety pupillary reactions return to normal

Diagnosis	Cause	Pupil	Comment
Horner's syndrome	Oculosympathetic palsy	Reactions to light and near are unimpaired; increased anisocoria in darkness (dilation insufficiency); miosis in the affected eye	Moderate ptosis; elevation of the lower lid; apparent enophthalmos; heterochromia of the iris may be present if the lesion is congenital or long-standing ($>10\,$yrs); diminished sweating on the ipsilateral part of the face if the lesion is pre-ganglionic
Horner's syndrome (preganglionic lesion)	Lesion between hypothalamus and C7–T2 (first neurone) or between the spinal cord and the superior cervical ganglion (second neurone)	As before	Possible causes are brain-stem ischaemia (Wallenberg's syndrome), thyroid disease or mediastinal mass
Horner's syndrome (postganglionic lesion)	Lesion along the third neurone which ascends along the internal carotid artery to enter the skull where it joins the ophthalmic division of the trigeminal nerve	As before	Most common underlying abnormalities of isolated postganglionic lesions are either idiopathic or associated with vascular headache syndromes (cluster headache) and are almost always benign

Diagnosis	Cause	Pupil	Comment
Argyll–Robertson pupil	Lesion to the Edinger–Westphal nucleus in its rostral area	Both pupils are small (although they may be asymmetrical); light–near dissociation	Underlying pathology is syphilis (rare since the advent of antibiotics); often wrongly diagnosed instead of tonic pupils (see below)
Aberrant regeneration of third nerve palsy	Synkinesis, e.g. posttraumatic	Pupillary constriction on innervation of the medial or internal rectus muscle or a different muscle	In contrast to Argyll–Robertson pupil, there is pupillary response not only to near stimulus but also to abduction
Tonic pupil	Mostly idiopathic, sometimes orbital disease or orbital trauma that affects the ciliary ganglion and causes denervation of its post-ganglionic fibres	Typically, in acute disease dilated pupil nonreactive to light and near vision, but constricts to 0.1% pilocarpine. In the further course of the disease, near reaction returns due to misdirected regeneration of accomodative fibres to the sphincter muscle.	Predominantly in young women; often associated with decreased jerk reflexes (Holmes–Adie syndrome)

EFFERENT PUPILLARY DISORDERS: DIAGNOSTIC ALGORITHM

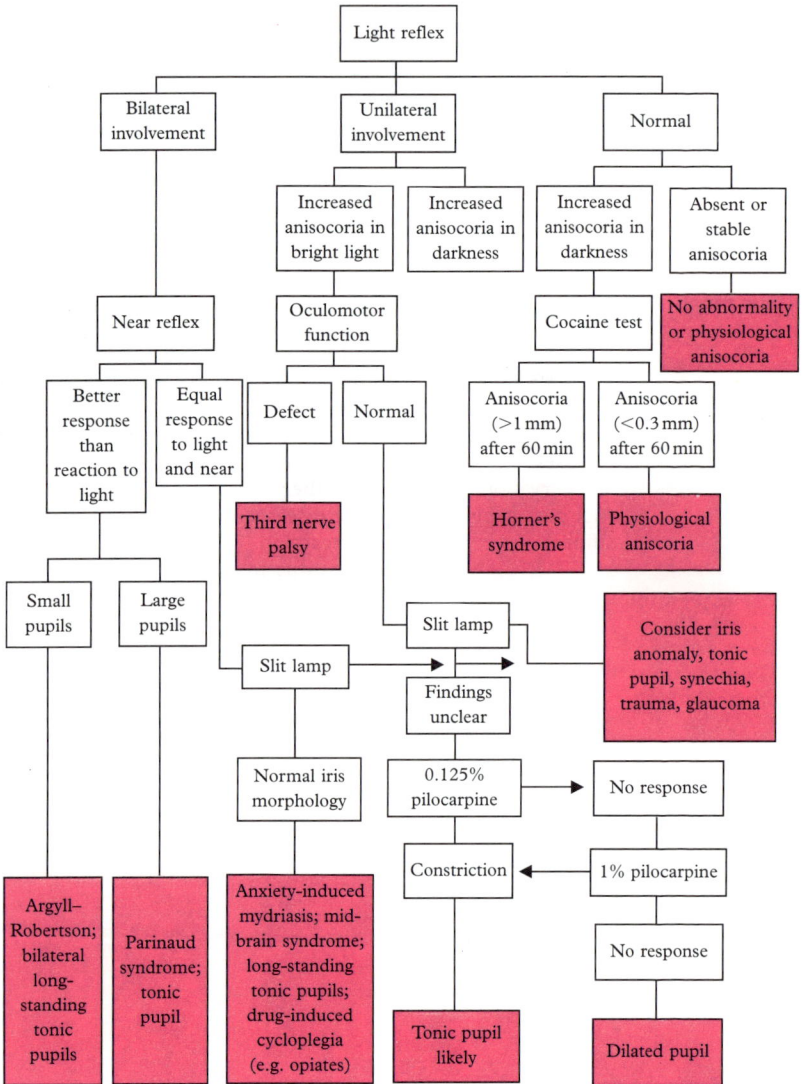

EFFERENT PUPILLARY DISORDERS: PHARMACOLOGICAL TESTS

Test	Indication	Mechanism	Normal response	Pathological response
0.125% pilocarpine	Tonic pupil	Demonstration of denervation hypersensitivity	No response	Constriction
1% pilocarpine	Drug-induced cycloplegia	Demonstration of muscarinic receptor blockade	Miosis	No response
5% cocaine	Confirms or excludes the presence or Horner's syndrome	Cocaine prevents the re-uptake of norepinephrine from the synaptic cleft	No anisocoria (both pupils dilate)	Anisocoria (difference between pupillary diameters >1 mm after 1 h)
1% hydroxyam-phetamine or 5% pholedrine	Differentiation between pre-ganglionic and post-ganglionic Horner's syndrome	Hydroxyam-phetamine releases endogenous noradreualine from a sympathetic endneuron	Both pupils dilate equally	In third-neurone Horner's syndrome the involved pupil dilates less than the normal one) whereas in preganglionic Horner's syndrome, both pupils will respond normally
Tropicamide–phenylephrine	To exclude a dilation malfunction	Parasympa-tholytic and sympathomi-metic stimulus	Mydriasis	Insufficient dilation due to iris lesions

DIFFERENTIAL DIAGNOSIS OF THE FIXED PUPIL

	Spontaneous appearance	With tropicamide	With cocaine	With pilocarpine
Paralytic mydriasis (oculomotor palsy)				
Spastic mydriasis (sympathetic stimulation)				
Spastic miosis (parasympathetic stimulation)				
Paralytic miosis (sympathetic palsy)				

HORNER'S SYNDROME

THE OCULOSYMPATHETIC PATHWAYS

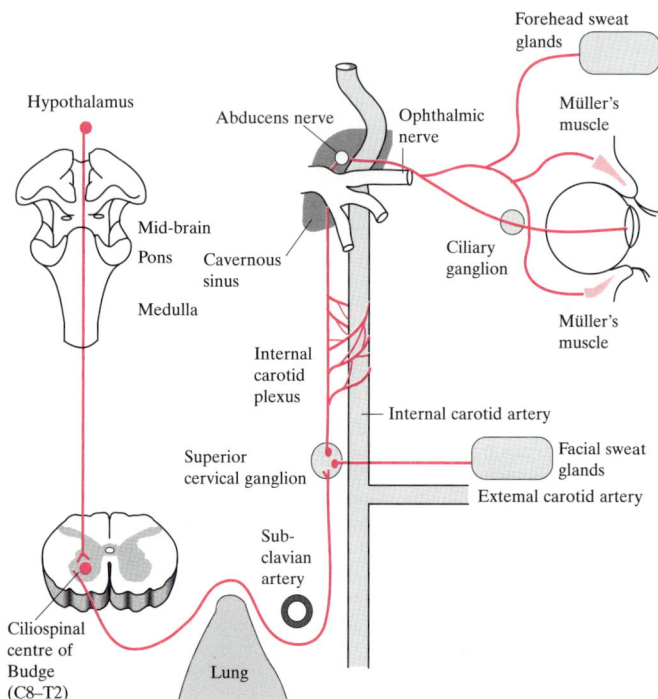

EFFECTS OF COCAINE AND HYDROXYAMPHETAMINE ON THE PUPILS IN HORNER'S SYNDROME

Test	Result	Interpretation
Cocaine to both eyes	Anisocoria (>1 mm after 1 h)	Horner's syndrome
	Bilateral dilation	Horner's syndrome excluded
Hydroxyamphetamine to both eyes	Absent or reduced response	Third-neurone Horner's syndrome
	Bilateral dilation	Preganglionic Horner's syndrome

Note:
- Bilateral dilation after hydroxyamphetamine test confirms preganglionic Horner's syndrome only if the cocaine test is abnormal. There is no indication for a hydroxyamphetamine test if the cocaine test is normal. Absent response confirms third-neurone Horner's syndrome (cocaine test unnecessary), but must confirm with phenylephrine that involved pupil able to dilate.
- There is no pharmacological test that can differentiate a first- and second-neurone Horner's syndrome. Although the presence of related neurological deficits in the first (such as after ischaemia of the brain-stem) often helps to distinguish it from the latter, first-neurone Horner's syndrome may be the only indication for a severe injury in the absence of other neurological signs.

AFFERENT PUPILLARY DISORDERS

RELATIVE AFFERENT PUPILLARY DISORDERS

1. Refractive error	Never
2. Unilateral occlusion	Temporary (contralateral)
3. Opaque media	Never (only exception: dense vitreous haemorrhage)
4. Marked anisocoria	Moderate (in the small pupil)
5. Amblyopia	Occasionally (mostly mild)
6. Macular disease	Only in asymmetrical cases
7. Unilateral optic nerve disease	Always
8. Chiasm lesion	Frequent
9. Optic tract lesion	Practically always (contralateral to the side of the lesion)
10. Retrogenicular lesion	Occasionally (lesion near the lateral geniculate body)

FURTHER INVESTIGATIONS IN PUPILLARY DEFECTS

Diagnosis	Investigations
Oculomotor palsy	Pupillary involvement indicates compression by a posterior communicating artery aneurysm (basilar aneurysms are a rare cause of third-nerve palsy); a suspected aneurysm always has to be excluded urgently (MRI, angiography); absent pupillary involvement indicates microangiopathy such as diabetes or hypertension affecting the blood vessels supplying the central part of the nerve, but sparing the superficial pupillary fibres; an oculomotor palsy may be associated with ipsilateral miosis, usually an indication for a cavernous sinus lesion compressing the sympathetic fibres accompanying the internal carotid artery to enter the cavernous sinus.
Tonic pupil	Tonic pupil has no long-term bad prognosis for life or vision. Patient should be told that it is harm less. In the presence of an underlying neuropathy (e.g. Sky-Drager syndrome), arrange for a neurological assessment.
Horner's syndrome in children	Cervical or mediastinal neuroblastoma should be suspected (unless there is a history of previous trauma).
Third-neurone Horner's syndrome	Postganglionic Horner's syndrome is either idiopathic or associated with vascular headache syndromes which are almost always benign. If other cranial nerve are involved, a mass must be suspected. If acute ouset, carotida dissection possible cause. MRI mandatory.
Preganglionic Horner's syndrome	Chest X-rays, medical and neurological work-up: MRI, if abnormal neurological opinion.

MYDRIATICS, CYCLOPLEGICS

Drug	Concentration	Maximum response	Duration of response
Atropine	0.5–2%	1.5–24 hours	3–12 days
Scopolamine	0.1–0.25%	40–90 minutes	6–72 hours
Homatropine	1%	50–80 minutes	6–48 hours
Tropicamide	0.5%	20–30 minutes	1–6 hours
Cyclopentolate	0.5–1%	30–60 minutes	8–36 hours
Phenylephrine	2.5–10%	30–60 minutes	4–12 hours
Pholedrine	5%	20–60 minutes	3–5 hours

PUPILLARY LIGHT RESPONSE IN THE COMATOSE PATIENT

EARLY STAGES OF THALAMIC COMPRESSION WITH EARLY HERNIATION (THALAMIC PUPILS)

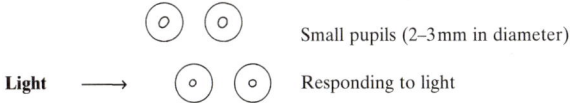

Small pupils (2–3mm in diameter)

Light ⟶ Responding to light

FOCAL DAMAGE AT THE PONTINE LEVEL OR OPIOID OVERDOSE (PINPOINT PUPILS)

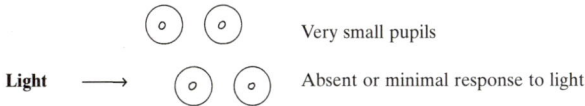

Very small pupils

Light ⟶ Absent or minimal response to light

DOWNWARD TRANSTENTORIAL HERNIATION AT THE MID-BRAIN LEVEL OR BELOW (FIXED DILATED PUPILS)

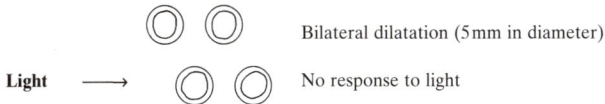

Bilateral dilatation (5mm in diameter)

Light ⟶ No response to light

Chapter 14

OCULAR DRUGS

LOCAL AND REGIONAL ANAESTHETICS

LOCAL ANAESTHETICS

Preparation	Concentration	Onset	Duration	Maximum dose
Lignocaine	0.5/1/2%	<2 min	60–90 min	200 mg
Lignocaine + adrenaline 1:200 000	0.5/1/2%	<2 min	90–120 min	500 mg
Mepivacaine	0.5/1/2%	<2 min	60–90 min	300 mg
Mepivacaine + adrenaline 1:200 000	0.5/1/2%	<2 min	60–90 min	500 mg
Bupivacaine	0.25/0.5/0.75%	10–20 min	60–150 min	150 mg
Bupivacaine + adrenaline 1:200 000	0.25/0.5/0.75%	10–20 min	60–150 min	150 mg

REGIONAL ANAESTHESIA

	Nerves	Indication	Application
Retrobulbar, peribulbar	II, III, (IV), V_1, (V_2), VI	Procedures on the globe	One-point injection (inferotemporal orbital quadrant) or two-point injection (inferotemporal and superonasal orbital quadrants)
Lid akinesia	VII	Optional supplement for retro- and peribulbar injections	To the region of the mandibular branch (O'Brien) or temporal and below the orbital rim (van Lint)
Supraorbital nerve	Supraorbital nerve, lacrimal nerve	Conjunctival, upper-lid, and forehead procedures	Supraorbital notch
Infra-orbital nerve	Infraorbital nerve	Lower-lid surgery and procedures on the medial canthus	Infraorbital foramen

Note: Most upper- and lower-lid procedures do not require lid akinesia and are undertaken under infiltration anaesthesia, e.g. Xylocaine 2% (lignocaine 20 mg/ml + adrenaline 1:200 000).

ANTIBIOTICS

CATEGORIES OF ANTIBIOTICS

Group	Subgroup	Derivatives
Penicillins		
Benzylpenicillin		Penicillin G
Oral penicillins	Phenoxymethylpenicillins	Penicillin V
Penicillinase-resistant penicillins	Isoxazolylpenicillins	Cloxacillin, flucloxacillin, temocillin
Broad-spectrum penicillins	Amoxybenzylpenicillins	Ampicillin, amoxycillin, bacampicillin
	Acylaminopenicillins	Azlocillin, piperacillin
	Carboxypenicillins	Ticarcillin
Cephalosporins		
Parenteral, limited penicillinase resistance	Cephazolin	Cephazolin
Orally active, limited penicillinase resistance	Cephalexin	Cephalexin, cefaclor, cefadroxil
Parenteral, increased penicillinase resistance	Cefuroxime	Cefuroxime, cephamandole
	Cefoxitin	Cefoxitin
	Cefotaxime	Cefotaxime, ceftriaxone, ceftizoxime
	Ceftazidime	Ceftazidime, cefpirome
Other β-lactam antibiotics	Monobactame	Aztreonam
	β-lactamase inhibitors	Clavulanic acid, tazobactam
Bacteriostatic broad-spectrum antibiotics	Tetracyclines	Tetracycline, doxycycline, minocycline
	Chloramphenicol	Chloramphenicol
Other antibiotics	Macrolides	Erythromycin, clarithromycin, azithromycin, spiramycin
	Polymyxins	Polymyxin B, colistin
	Lincosamides	Clindamycin
	Glycopeptides	Vancomycin, teicoplanin
Sulphonamides		Sulphadiazine, sulphamethoxazole
Sulphamethoxazole and trimethoprim		Co-trimoxzole
Nitroimidazole		Metronidazole, tinidazole
Aminoglycosides	Old aminoglycosides	Streptomycin, neomycin, kanamycin
	New aminoglycosides	Gentamicin, tobramycin, netilmicin, amikacin
4-Quinolones		Norfloxacin, ofloxacin, ciprofloxacin

ANTIBIOTICS, *cont.*

MECHANISM OF ANTIBACTERIAL ACTION

Antibiotic	Action Site	Action Mechanism	Action Effect
β-lactam antibiotics (penicillins, cephalosporins)	Cell wall	Muramine acid synthesis	Bactericidal
Fosfomycin		Pyruvic transferase	
Chloramphenicol	Ribosome	Peptidic transferase	Bacteriostatic
Tetracycline		Ribosome A	
Macrolides (erythromycin)		Translocation	
Clindamycin		Peptidic transferase (?)	
Fusidic acid		Elongation factor G	
Aminoglycosides		Catalytic enzymes	Bactericidal
Rifampicin	Nucleic acid	RNA polymerase	Bactericidal
Nitroimidazole		DNA strands	
Polymyxins	Cell membrane	Phospholipids	Bactericidal
Amphotericin B		Ergosterol synthesis	Fungiostatic
Sulphonamides	Folate synthesis	Pteroate synthesis	Bacteriostatic
Trimethoprim		Dihydrofolate reductase	

ANTIBACTERIAL SPECTRUM OF PENICILLINS

	Penicillin G, Penicillin V	Flucloxacillin	Amoxycillin	Azlocillin, Piperacillin	Co-amoxiclav (amoxycillin + clavulanic acid)
Enterococci	∅	∅	++	++	++
Haemophilus	∅	∅	++	++	++
Klebsiella	∅	∅	∅	∅	+
Pneumococci, streptococci	++	++	++	++	++
Proteus mirabilis	∅	∅	++	++	++
Proteus vulgaris	∅	∅	∅	++	+
Pseudomonas aeruginosa	∅	∅	∅	++	∅
Penicillinase-producing staphylococci	∅	++	∅	∅	++
Staphylococci	++	++	++	+	++

Interpretation of symbols:

++ = very effective (main indication in red)

+ = effective

∅ = not effective

ANTIBIOTICS, *cont.*

DAILY DOSES OF ANTIBIOTICS

Antibiotic	Route of administration	Adult	Child (neonates excluded)
Penicillin G	i.v., i.m.	1–5 (maximum 20) million IU	0.05–0.5 (maximum 1) million IU/kg
Penicillin V	oral	1–5 (maximum 20) million IU	0.05 (maximum 0.1) million IU/kg
Flucloxacillin	oral, i.v.	1.8–3.6 million IU 2–4 g (maximum 10)	50 mg/kg (maximum 100)
Ampicillin	i.v.	3–6 g (maximum 20)	100 mg/kg (maximum 200–400)
Amoxycillin	oral	1–1.5 g (maximum 3)	50 mg/kg
Azlocillin	i.v.	6 g (maximum 20)	3 × 75 mg/kg
Cephazolin	i.v.	2–6 g	50 mg/kg
Cefoxitin	i.v.	3–6 g	60 mg/kg (maximum 150)
Cefotaxime, Ceftazidime	i.v.	3–6 g	50 mg/kg (maximum 150)
Ceftriaxone	i.v.	1–2 g (maximum 4)	30–60 mg/kg
Cefaclor, Cefadroxil	oral	1.5–3 g	30–50 mg/kg
Cefixime	oral	400 mg	8 mg/kg
Cefuroxime axetil	oral	0.5–1 g	20–30 mg/kg
Cefpodoxime	oral	400 mg	–
Imipenem	i.v.	1.5–2 g (maximum 4)	3–60 mg/kg
Aztreonam	i.v.	2–6 g (maximum 8)	45–90 mg/kg (maximum 120)
Co-amoxiclav	oral	750/375 mg– 1.5/1.125 g	750/186 mg–1.5/ 0.558 g (>6 years)
	i.v.	3/0.6–4/0.8 g	25/5 mg/kg– 75/15 mg/kg (>3 months)
Gentamicin, Tobramycin	i.v.	2–3 mg/kg (maximum 5)	3–5 mg/kg
Amikacin	i.v.	1 g	15 mg/kg
Spectinomycin	i.m.	2 g (one dose)	–
Doxycycline	oral, i.v.	100–200 mg	2–4 mg/kg
Erythromycin	oral, i.v.	1–2 g	30–50 mg/kg
Clarithromycin	oral	0.5–1 g	–
Fusidic acid	oral	1.5 g (maximum 3)	20 mg/kg
Vancomycin	i.v.	2 g	40 mg/kg
Clindamycin	oral, i.v.	0.6–1.8 g	10–20 mg/kg
Metronidazole	oral, i.v.	1–1.5 g	20–30 mg/kg

Antibiotic	Route of administration	Adult	Child (neonates excluded)
Rifampicin	oral, i.v.	0.6 g	10 mg/kg
Fosfomycin	i.v.	6–15 g	100–200 mg/kg
Chloramphenicol	oral, i.v.	2 g	50 mg/kg (maximum 80)
Ofloxacin	oral, i.v.	400–800 mg	–
Ciprofloxacin	oral	0.5–1.5 g	–
	i.v.	400–800 mg	–
Norfloxacin	oral	400–800 mg	–
Co-trimoxazole	oral	1.6 g (sulphamethoxazole)	30 mg/kg (sulphamethoxazole)
Trimethoprim	oral	400 mg	6 mg/kg

ANTIBIOTIC SENSITIVITY

Organism	Penicillin G	Ampicillin	Cephazolin	Cefoxitin	Ceftriaxone	Imipenem	Gentamicin	Doxycycline	Erythromycin	Clindamycin	Ciprofloxacin	Co-trimoxazole
Acinetobacter	–	–	–	–	±	+	+	±	–	–	++	–
Actinomyces israelii	++	+	+	+	+	+	–	+	+	+	±	+
Aeromonas hydrophilia	–	–	–	+	+	+	+	+	–	–	++	+
Bacillus anthracis	++	+	+	+	+	+	+	+	+	+	+	+
Bacteroides fragilis				+		++		±	±	++		±
Bordetella pertussis	–	+	–	–	–	–	–	++	++	–	+	+
Borrelia burgdorferi	++	+	+	+	++	+	–	+	+	–	–	–
Borrelia recurrentis	+	+	+	+	+	+	–	++	+	–	–	+
Brucella	–	–	–	–	–	–	+	++	–	–	+	–
Campylobacter jejuni	–	+	–	–	±	+	+	+	++	–	+	–
Clamydia	–	–	–	–	–	–	–	++	++	–	±	+
Citrobacter	–	–	–	–	±	+	++	+	–	–	+	+
Clostridia	++	±	±	±	±	+		+	+	±	±	
Corynebacterium diphtheriae	++	+	+	+	+	+	+	+	+	+	+	–

ANTIBIOTIC SENSITIVITY, *cont.*

Organism	Penicillin G	Ampicillin	Cephazolin	Cefoxitin	Ceftriaxone	Imipenem	Gentamicin	Doxycycline	Erythromycin	Clindamycin	Ciprofloxacin	Co-trimoxazole
Erysipelothrix rhusiopathiae	++	+	+	+	+	+	−	+	+	+	+	+
Francisella tularensis	−	−	−	−	−	−	++	++	−	−	−	−
Fusobacteria	++	+	+	+	+	+	−	+	−	++	+	+
Haemophilus ducreyi	−	+	+	+	+	−	−	+	+	−	++	++
Haemophilus influenzae	−	+	+	+	++	+	±	++	±	−	++	+
Klebsiella	−	−	±	++	++	++	++	+	−	−	++	++
Legionella	−	−	−	−	+	+	−	+	++	−	+	−
Leptospira	++	+	+	+	+	+	−	++	−	−	−	−
Listeria	+	++	−	−	−	+	±	+	+	+	+	+
Moraxella	−	−	+	+	++	++	+	++	±	−	+	+
Nocardia asteroides	−	−	−	−	+	+	−	+	−	+	−	++
Pasteurella multocida	++	+	+	+	+	+	+	++	+	−	+	+
Pneumococci	++	+	±	±	±	+		±	+	+	±	
Pseudomonas cepacia	−	−	−	−	−	−	−	−	−	−	+	+
Pseudomonas mallei	−	−	−	−	−	−	+	++	−	−	+	+
Pseudomonas pseudomallei	−	−	−	−	−	−	−	+	−	−	+	+
Rickettsia	−	−	−	−	−	−	−	++	+	−	+	−
Salmonella	−	+	−	−	++	+	−	−	−	−	++	++
Serratia marcescens	−	−	−	±	++	++	+	−	−	−	+	±
Staphylococcus aureus	+	±	++	+	±	+	±	±	+	++	+	±
Staphylococcus epidermidis	−	−	+	±	±	+	±	−	±	++	+	−
Streptococci	++	±	±	±	±	+	±	±	+	+	±	±
Xanthomonas maltophilia	−	−	−	−	−	−	−	+	−	−	±	+
Yersinia	−	−	−	−	+	+	+	+	−	−	++	++

Interpretation of symbols:

++ = very effective, treatment of choice ± = variable effectiveness
+ = effective, some disadvantages, second choice − = not effective

SYSTEMIC CORTICOSTEROID THERAPY

SIDE-EFFECTS OF GLUCOCORTICOID THERAPY

Endocrine system	Reduced glucose tolerance, diabetes mellitus Cushing's syndrome Adrenal suppression Suppression of growth in children Amenorrhoea, hirsutism, impotence
Electrolytes	Hypokalaemia Sodium retention with oedema Hypercalciuria
Skeletal and muscular system	Osteoporosis Aseptic bone necrosis Muscle wasting
Skin	Striae Acne Delayed healing
Eyes	Elevated intraocular pressure (does not occur prior to 2–4 weeks after commencement of treatment: 30% of the population respond with mild elevation of IOP, 5% are high responders with markedly raised IOP) Cataract
Mental disturbances	Depression, euphoria, psychosis
Gastrointestinal system	Peptic ulceration Pancreatitis
Circulation	Hypertension Thrombosis

PREDNISOLONE THERAPY

Commencement of treatment

High-dose bolus	250 mg to maximum 1 g
High-dose therapy	Initial dose 80–100 mg (maximum 250 mg)
Low-dose therapy	Initial dose 7.5–40 mg

Maintenance

Range of dosage
>10 mg prednisolone
<10 mg prednisolone
<7 mg prednisolone
Low-dosage maintenance
  therapy

Dosage reduction
To be tapered off by 5 mg per week
To be tapered off by 1 mg every 1–2 weeks
To be tapered off by 0.5–1 mg every 4 weeks
2.5–15 mg prednisolone daily

Application

Circadian therapy   Complete daily dosage to be given in the morning

Alternating therapy   Double dose every other day (less adrenal suppression and suppression of growth in children than in daily application; alternating therapy is not suitable for severe acute disease)

Long-term prednisolone therapy

Every month   Enquire: abdominal pain, back pain, infections?
Check: cushingoid habitus and facies, blood pressure, blood in faeces

Every 3 months   Check: erythrocyle sedimentation rate, full blood count, blood lipids, glycosuria, electrolytes
Slit lamp: IOP, clarity of the lens

Every 6 months   Check: bone density, chest X-ray
In gastrointestinal complaints, arrange for gastroscopy

Chapter 15

HISTORY OF OPHTHALMOLOGY

1700 BC

'The fee for the treatment of an ocular abscess with a knife amounts to 10 silver shekels, two silver shekels if the patient is a slave. If the physician kills the patient or blinds him by using a blunt knife, then his hand is to be amputated' (from the oldest medical law, the Codex Hammurabi, with reference to eye surgery).

1500 BC

The most comprehensive source of Egyptian medicine is the long papyrus, acquired by **Georg Ebers** in 1872 and named after him. It reports on 100 various eye diseases and their treatment.

Circa 150 AD

Two ophthalmic manuscripts 'Optics' and 'Diagnostics of Eye Diseases' were written by the Greek physician **Galen** (130–201). Unfortunately, they were both lost.

1267

'Opus Majus' was published by the English scientist, philosopher and Franciscan monk **Roger Bacon** (1214–1292). It mentions convex glass as a useful tool for old people and subjects with weak eyes. This observation contains the idea of lenses for optical correction. In the 15th century, there were already two types of spectacle lenses – biconvex convergent lenses and biconcave divergent lenses.

Circa 1600

Modern optics was founded in the 16th century. The astronomer **Johannes Kepler** (1571–1630) wrote his work 'Dioptrik', and the Jesuit **Christoph Scheiner** (1575–1650) published his work 'Fundamentum Opticum'. **Leeuwenhoek** (1632–1723) designed the first functional microscope.

Circa 1620

Snell's law was introduced by the Dutch physicist **Willebord Snell** (1591–1626).

Circa 1700

Cataract was explained by **Pierre Brisseau** as a clouding of the crystalline lens.

1707

The first documented cataract extraction was performed by the Frenchman **Saint-Yves** (1667–1736). Using a corneal incision, he removed a cataractous lens which had dislocated in the anterior chamber.

1752

Extracapsular cataract extraction was introduced by the Frenchman **Jacques Daviel** (1689–1762).

1762

Jacques Daviel was offered the first chair of ophthalmology at the University of Paris but he died shortly before the nomination took place, and the professorial chair was cancelled due to the mediocre qualities of his successor.

Early 19th century

Ophthalmology developed into a surgical speciality. Eye clinics were started in 1805 by **Joseph Beer** in Vienna and **John C. Saunders** in the UK.

Mid-19th century

The method of direct opthalmoscopy was published by the physicist and physiologist **Hermann von Helmholtz** (1821–1894). Shortly after, in 1852, indirect ophthalmoscopy was presented by **Christian Reute** (1810–1867). **Richard Förster** (1825–1902) developed the concept of perimetry.

1828–1870

Albrecht von Graefe, a professor in Berlin, introduced the iridectomy, improved cataract surgery and developed new methods for correction of strabismus. During his brief 19 years of surgical work he performed 10 000 cataract operations.

1864

Refractive errors, accommodation and the effect of hypermetropia on convergent squint are described in 'Die Anomalien der Refraktion und Akkommodation des Auges' by **Frans C. Donders** (1818–1889).

1877

The beneficial effect of the alkaloid physostigmine on elevated intraocular pressure was discovered by **L. Laraquer.**

Circa 1880

The first internationally accepted ophthalmic textbook 'Handbuch der Ophthalmologie' was written by **Alfred Graefe**, his cousin **Albrecht von Graefe** and **Edwin Theodor Saemisch.**

1884

Cocaine was introduced as a local anaesthetic by **Carl Koller**.

1906

The first successful keratoplasty was carried out by **Eduard Zirn** (1863–1944).

1911

The slit lamp was introduced by the Swedish ophthalmologist **Allvar G. Gullstrand** (1862–1930). He was awarded the Nobel Prize in 1911 for his experiments on the refraction of light in the eye.

1916

Thermocautery for retinal detachment repair was introduced by the Swiss **Jules G. Gonin** (1870–1935).

1921

'Atlas der Spaltlampenmikroskopie des lebenden Auges' [Atlas of Slit Lamp Microscopy of the Living Eye] was published by **Alfred Vogt**.

1871–1940

The German **Alfred Bielschowsky**, one of the most significant strabologists and head of the ophthalmic department in Marburg (1912) and later in Breslau (1923), was forced to leave his position in 1934 because of his Jewish origin. He emigrated to the USA in 1936 to become director of the Dartmouth Eye Institute in Hanover, New Hampshire.

1929

An orthoptic training school was opened in London in 1930 by **Mary Maddox** with the support of her father, **Ernest Maddox**, an ophthalmologist in Edinburgh, and **Sheila Mayou**.

1946

Photocoagulation, initially with sunlight, was introduced by the German **Gerd Meyer-Schwickerath** (1920–1992).

1948

Scleral buckling for closure of retinal breaks was introduced by **Ernst Custodis** (1898–1990).

1948

The first artificial intraocular lens was implanted in a human eye by **H. Ridley** at St Thomas' Hospital in London.

1960

Fluorescein angiography was introduced by two American medical students, **Harald Novotny** and **David Alvis**.

1950s and 1960s

Intracapsular cataract extraction was improved by **Barraquer** in 1958 (fermentative zonulolysis) and by **Krwawicz** in 1961 (cryo-extraction). At the same time, however, extracapsular cataract extraction was reintroduced. **Kelman** presented the phaco-emulsification procedure in 1967.

1968

Argon laser for retinal photocoagulation was first used by **Francois L'Esperance** in New York. The first commercial argon laser coagulator was built in 1970.

1986

First clinical use of a photo-ablative excimer laser by **Theo Seiler** and **Josef Wollensak** in Berlin.

SYNDROMES AND RARE DISEASES

Abbreviations for modes of inheritance:– AD = autosomal dominant; AR = autosomal recessive; X-chromosomal; XR = X-chromosomal recessive.

Abetalipoproteinemia: Bassen-Kornzweig syndrome.

Abt-Letterer-Siwe disease: Histiocytosis X.

Adie's syndrome: Pupillotonia and abnormal muscle proprioceptor reflexes. Usually harmless. Aetiology unclear.

Aicardi's syndrome: Jack-knife salaam seizures in early childhood, agenesis of the corpus callosum and foci of peripapillary lacunar chorioretinopathy. Occurs only in girls. Male fetuses, which only have abnormal X-chromosome, die *in utero*. Often there are costovertebral malformations, severe psychomotor retardation and hypotonic tetra- or diplegias. There may be additional ocular anomalies: microphthalmus, hypoplasia and coloboma of the optic nerve, retinal vessel anomalies, iris synechiae, persistent pupillary membrane, ptosis, strabismus and nystagmus.

AIDS (acquired immune deficiency syndrome): HIV (human immunodeficiency virus) causes disorders of the cellular immune system, with marked reduction in the number of T-helper cells. Susceptibility to oportunistic infections and predisposition to Kaposi's sarcoma and malignant non-Hodgkin lymphomas. Ophthalmological features: microangiopathy syndrome, chorioretinitis, neoplasm, neuro-ophthalmological abnormalities.

Alagille's syndrome (arteriohepatic dysplasia): Characteristic features are intrahepatic biliary hypoplasia with jaundice, pulmonary stenosis, typical facies and growth retardation. Ophthalmological findings are posterior embryotoxon, Axenfeld or Rieger anomalies, keratotonus, corectopia, cataract, retinal changes, optic nerve anomalies, microphthalmos with strabismus.

Aland island disease (Forsius-Eriksson disease): Fundal hypopigmentation, foveal hypoplasia, myopia, astigmatism, nystagmus. A form of congenital stationary night-blindness (CNSB) with abnormal ERG indicating rod and cone dystrophy.

Albinism: (I) oculocutaneous: AR. a) Tyrosinase-negative (complete albinims): white hair, 0.1 vision; b) tyrosinase-positive (incomplete albinism): vision reduced to varying degree. **(II) ocular:** AR or XR; affects only eyes, nystagmus, sensitivity to light, vision usually better than 0.1; minor defects of iris pigmentation. Crossing anomalies of the optic nerve fibres in the chiamsa can be found in all forms.

Alport's syndrome: Genetically heterogeneous syndrome (AD – recessive or X-chromosomal). Disorders of the basal membrane caused by collagen defects. Familial nephritis, inner-ear deafness, anterior lenticonus, spherophakia or cataract (cortex).

Alström's syndrome: Atypical retinal dystrophy, obesity, inner-ear deafness, diabetes mellitus.

Amebic keratitis: Typical features are history of wearing contact lenses and of corneal perineuritis, causing severe pain which often seem to bear no relationship to the findings. In the further course circular infiltrates will form, often with bacterial hyperinfection and hypopyon formation.

Amyloidosis: Term given to a group of etiologically distinct diseases, which have the deposition of amyloid fibrils (glycoproteins) in common. In familial inherited polyneuropathic amyloidosis, a form of systemic amyloidosis, there are often deposits in the vitreous. Ocular amyloidosis is the localized form.

Angiomatosis retinae: Hippel-Lindau syndrome.

Apert's syndrome (acrocephalosyndactily syndrome): Skeletal dysplasia with changes largely in the skull region and the distal parts of the limbs.

Argyll-Robertson phenomenon: Fixed pupil as part of syphilitic disease (tabes dorsalis).

Arnold-Chiari syndrome: Chiari syndrome.

Ataxia teleangiectasia: Louis Bar's syndrome.

Atrophia gyrate: AR-inherited metabolic disorder (hyperornithinemia) characterized by large, arc-like areas of chorioretinal atrophy in the middle and outer parts of the fundal periphery. Affected areas expand and become confluent. Manifests itself in the 2nd to 3rd decade. A cataract (posterior subcapsular clouding) can additionally impair vision.

Autosomal dominant optic atrophy: Usually as mild form, beginning in early childhood. Never ends in blindness, but vision may decrease to 0.1 in the 5th decade. Vision between 0.2 and 0.6 is typical, as is abnormal blue-color perception (if vision < 0.5). With increasing loss of function abnormal red-green perception occurs. Depending on the loss of function, changes in the optic disc may vary from pallor on its temporal aspect to complete optic nerve atrophy and central, paracentral or centrocecal scotoma. Optical atrophy is always bilateral. A family history should be obtained.

Axenfeld's anomaly: Iridotrabeculocorneal dysgenesis. NB: A posterior embryotoxon can be found in 15% of all *normal* eyes.

Balints syndrome: Cognitive visual disorder. Independent of the quality of visual acuity and the visual field, the patient can only perceive part of an image (simultaneous agnosia). It occurs in bilateral lesions of the upper occipital lobe.

Bardet-Biedl syndrome: Clinical signs are retinitis pigmentosa (RP), obesity and small stature, poly- and syndactyly. Hypogenitalism and frequently associated with nephrophthisis or interstitial nephritis. Oligophrenia may occur. RP becomes symptomatic in the 1st decade. Molecular genetic tests show genetic heterogeneity. Laurence-Moon syndrome (hypogenitalism, RP, spastic paraplegia, mental retardation) is a special form and not a separate entity. Cf. RP associated syndrome.

Bassen-Kornzweig syndrome: Abetalipoproteinemia with retinitis pigmentosa (cf. RP associated syndrome). Insufficient or missing formation of alipoprotein B and deficient (type II, homozygous, AR) or absent (type I, heterozygous, AR) betalipoprotein. LDL fraction decreased or absent in lipid-electrophoresis, serum vitamin E reduced. Fat malabsorption, steotorrhea and akanthocytosis are present from birth. Cerebral ataxia and sensorimotor neuropathy follow during the 1st decade. The symptoms can be ameliorated by high-dosage vitamin A and E.

Batten's disease: Neuronal ceroid-lipofuscinosis.

Bechterew's disease (ankylosing spondyloarthritis [AS]): Chronic inflammatory rheumatic disease predominantly of the vertebrae. Commonly starting in the sacroiliac joints, it extends to cervical and thoracic vertebrae. Associated with HLA-B27 antigen in 90% of cases. M : F = 10 : 1. Involvement of the eyes in about 30% of cases: (fibrinous) iridocyclitis. Ocular signs may precede the full picture of AS by 10–15 years.

Behçet's syndrome: Probably viral, autoimmune disease with widely distributed aphthous ulcers in the mouth, stomach, intestine and genitals. Cardinal manifestations: a) painful oral ulcers (in 99%); b) genital ulcers (in ca. 80%); c) eye involvement (in 80%): most often acute iridocyclitis, if first attack, possibly as hypopyoniritis; uveoretinitis; conjunctivitis and episcleritis. Other findings: cutaneous changes, arthritis (knee or ankle), CNS involvement, gastroenteritis, thrombophlebitis. Histologically, occlusive vasculitis. Common in China and Japan, also eastern Mediterranean (take careful history!). HLA-B5 may be demonstrated.

Behr's syndrome: AR. Optic nerve atrophy with CNS symptoms (mental retardation, ataxia, spaxticity, etc). Probably heterogeneous group of diseases with similar clinical picture.

Benedict's (nucleus ruber) syndrome: Focal oculomotor paresis and contralateral hemiparesis with rigor and intention tremor.

Best's maculopath (vitelliform macular atrophy): Macular atrophy with typical ophthalmological findings; early EOG abnormalities; later, decreasing vision.

Bloch-Sulzberger syndrome: Incontinentia pigmenti.

Boeck's disease: Sarcoidosis.

Botulism: Disease caused by the action of a toxin on cholinergic synapses after ingestion of spoilt tinned food or badly preserved meat and fish products. Botulinus toxin is formed by Colstridium botulinum in anerobic conditions. Due to the blocking of acetylcholine liberation, accomodation is disturbed. Eventually mydriasis, double vision, ptosis, paresis of the skeletal muscles and respiratory paralysis occur, as well as autonomic nervous system symptoms such as dry mouth, abnormal gastrointestinal motility and cardiac arrhythmias.

Bourneville-Pringle disease: tuberous sclerosis.

Brown's syndrome (superior oblique contracture): persistent impairment of upward gaze in adduction, caused by a too short tendon (congenital or postoperative) or a too tight tendon sheath. Contrary to the very rare isolated paresis of the inferior oblique muscle, passive motion is reduced (traction test with a pair of forceps). Also, in contrast to inferior oblique paresis, there is divergence on upward gazing (in adduction).

Butterfly dystrophy: AD. Macular dystrophy with continuing good vision. Abnormal EOG.

Canthaxanthine deposition in the retina: The carotinoid canthaxanthine is used as a protective medication in light dermatitis and also as a tanning agent. It can cause reversible crystalline deposits which are usually located around the macula. Definite amd persisting retinal lesions do not occur.

CAPE dystrophy (central areolar pigment epithelial dystrophy): AD. Normal ERG and EOG. Relatively good vision; abnormality of pigment epithelium more likely temporal of the fovea.

Carbohydrate-deficient glycoprotein (CDG) syndrome: Congenital liver disease, mental retardation and neurological impairment, usually inherited as AR. Frequently tapetoretinal degeneration and esotropia of early childhood.

Carotid sinus to cavernous sinus fistula: Defect in the arterial wall between carotid artery and cavernous sinus. Caused by trauma (high-flow shunt common) or spontaneously (atherosclerosis) (low-flow shunt common) or aneurysm. Symptoms usually prolonged, even if traumatic cause. Swelling of eye-lids with blue discoloration, pulsating exophthalmos. Flow murmur over the orbit (also perceived by patient), epibulbar congestion, glaucoma due to increased episcleral flow pressure. If low-flow shunt, symptoms correspondingly less marked (no pulsating exophthalmos).

Cat's eye syndrome: Partial trisomy 22q11. Anal atresia, coloboma, periauricular skin tags or fistulas.

Cerebrotendinous xanthomatosis: Storage disease: increased serum cholesterol concentration, cataract, xanthomatous swelling of tendons.

Chagas' disease (American trypanosomiasis): Most common tropical disease in South America. Caused by the single-cell parasite Trypanozoma cruzi. Transmission by rubbing of infected feces of a blood-sucking triatomine bug into the bite wound. In about 90% of cases the eye is the portal of entry. As a result, in ca. 10% of cases the acute clinical picture (Romana sign) consists of (usually unilateral) conjunctivitis and lid edema as well as regional lymphadenopathy. In 20% of infected cases complications of chronic Chagas' disease develop after an interval of decades and are due to a toxic/allergic damage of nervous tissue (neurotoxin, intramural plexus), resulting in major gastrointestinal lesions and dilated cardiomyopathy.

Chandler's syndrome: iridocorneoendothelial dystrophy.

CHARGE association: Malformation/retardation syndrome with multiple but characteristic symptoms: **c**oloboma, **h**eart defect, (choanal) **a**tresia, (mental) **r**etardation, **g**enital hypoplasia and **e**ar malformations. At least four of these must be present to make the diagnosis.

Charles Bonnet's syndrome: Visual hallucination with normal level of consciousness. Most of the patients will have visual impairment by an eye disease.

Charlin's syndrome: Unilateral paroxysmal conjunctival reddening, tears, rhinorrhea, neuralgia of the inner lid angle. Probably caused by neuralgia of the nasociliary nerve. Cf. Sluder's syndrome.

Chediak-Higashi syndrome: AR inheritance. Abnormality of lysosomes (impairment of membrane fusion), hypopigmentation (albinism) with photophobia.

Chiari's syndrome: Craniospinal maldevelopment with herniation of the cerebellum and medulla oblongata through the foramen magnum (f.m.) into the spinal canal. Type 1: caudal displacement of cerebellar tonsils through the f.m. into the spinal canal; type 2 (Arnold-Chiari syndrome): additional herniation of the brain-stem. Causes obstructive hydrocephalus, ataxia, nystagmus and compression of the brain-stem, spinal cord and cranial nerves; type 3: cervical meningomyelocele in addition to the other lesions.

Chiasma syndrome: Collective term given to abnormalities in the chiasma-sella region. Visual field disturbances (bitemporal hemianopsia), papilledema, optic nerve atropy, radiologically demonstrable sella changes and, in some cases, symptoms of hypophseal insufficiency. Most common causes are hypophyseal tumor, craniopharyngioma and meningioma.

Choroideremia, X-chromosomal recessive: Tapetochoroidal dystrophy with (later) atrophy of the choroid, pigment epithelium and of the photoreceptors. In the early stages there are localized atrophies, especially peripapillary and in the middle periphery, of pigment epithelium and of the choroid capillaries. These changes may be mistaken for the much rarer atrophia gyrata. As the macula remains unaffected for a relatively long time, the clinical course corresponds largely with that of retinitis pigmentosa (RP). There is early impairment in the ERG and EOG. In affected males the hyperpigmentation may make the differentiaition from RP very difficult. Of importance is the absence of bony spicules and the presence of spotty atrophies of choroicapillaries. Examination of the mother will be of help, because female carriers of the gene for choroideremia, in contrast to those with X-chromosomal RP, more frequently have fundal changes and more rarely reduced responses in the ERG.

Chronic progressive external opthalmoplegia (CPEO; Graefe's ophthalmoplegia): Degenerative ocular myopathy. Increasing ptosis and immobility of both eyes will develop over many years. Saccadic velocity is reduced. *No* abnormal pupils. Because the condition affects both eyes, strabismus is rare. If several organ system are affected, the term 'ophthalmoplegia plus' is used. The Kearn-Sayre syndrome, in which there is the full picture of generalized mitochondrial abnormality, is a special form.

CINCA syndrome (chronic infantile neurological cutaneous and articular s.): Chronic inflammatory disease with onset in childhood. Skin rash is the first symptom. Arthritis of the distal large joints, meningitis, growth retardation, deafness, keratitis, uveitis and papilledema follow.

Clival edge syndrome: Transient or permanent, partial or complete oculomotor paresis caused by the nerve being pressed against the clivus or by stretching of this nerve segment.

Cluster headache: Attacks of headache of usually sudden onset, commonly one to three times daily, often at night on waking up. Attacks generally last for 30–90 min; unbearable intensity, maximally over the orbits, strictly unilateral. May develop Horner's syndrome. Lacrimation, conjunctival injection, rhinorrhea. 80% of patients are men. It follows a sporadic course, with runs of seperate attacks (hence 'cluster').

Coats' disease: Vascular disease of retinal arteries with aneurysms (due to loss of pericytes), sometimes tumor-like exudations (due to loss of endothelial cells) and vascular occlusions (due to thickening of basal membrane), but practically never neovascularization. Unilateral in 90%. Severe forms predominantly in children and adolescents.

Cockayne's syndrome: Hereditary (AR) disease with ataxia, dwarfism, microcephaly, mental retardation, inner-ear deafness. Ocular signs: pigmented retinal degeneration (salt-and-pepper fundus), cataract (in ca. 25%), corneal ulcers or clouding, nystagmus and hypoplastic irises as well as irregular pupils.

Cogan's syndrome (I): Autoimmune disease affecting primarily corneal and vestibulocochlear organ. Typical eye involvement is bilateral stromakeratitis. But other ocular inflammatory manifestation also occur: episcleritis, scleritis, vasculitis or anterior uveitis. Fever, headache and joint pains are often associated with it. High risk of complete deafness, despite immunosuppressive treatment.

Cogan's syndrome (II): Oculomotor apraxia.

Cogan-Reese syndrome: iridoendothelial dystrophy.

Cohen's syndrome: AR inheritance. Mental retardation, striking facies (signs of oral dysmorphism), obesity of the trunk, muscular hypotonia. Often ocular changes: retinal and choroidal dystrophy, errors of refraction, coloboma formation, microphthalmos.

Cone-rod dystrophy: Photophobia, abnormal color sense and reduced visual acuity in the 1st or 2nd decade. ERG shows marked impairment of response by the rod system. As the photophobia increases, abnormal rod function can also be demonstrated. Early functional changes of the rod–dominated pigment epithelium/photoreceptor response in the EOG as well as oscillatory potentials in the ERG can be demonstrated. The main defect is assumed to be in the pigment epithelium or rod system. All kinds of mendelian inheritance have been observed. RP-associated syndromes may commonly occur with cone-rod dystrophy.

Congenital stationary night blindness (CSNB): Group of diseases which must be distinguished from the progressive forms of night blindness (retinitis pigmentosa). Typical shared characteristics: symptoms from birth, non-progressing course, largely intact outer borders on Goldmann perimetry. Frequently positive family history with XR, AD or AR inheritance pattern and characteristic findings in the ERG and dark adaptation measurements.
  - Forms with unremarkable fundus (mutations in rhodopsin gene: **Schubert-Bornschein type:** negative ERG. **Riggs type:** no negative ERG.
  - With fundus changes: **Albipunctate fundus with nyctalopia:** numerous small, sharply circumscribed spots, deep in the retina, at the posterior pole but excluding the macular region. **Oguchi's disease:** Metallic greyish white fundal reflex which after some time and in the dark becomes completely normal (Mizuo phenomenon). Cause of this disease, especially common among Japanese, is a mutation in the arrestin gene (chromosome 2q).

(Cornelia) de Lange's syndrome: Malformation-retardation syndrome with characteristic features: growth retardation, microcephaly, prominent eyebrow ridges, long and curved eyelashes.

Criswick-Schepens syndrome: Familial exudative vitreoretinopathy.

Crohn's disease: Autoimmune, chronic granulomatous inflammation of the intestinal tract. Often occurs in the small intestine (terminal ileitis), prone to segmental intestinal involvement (regional enteritis). Complications occur as result of perforation, chronic abscess and/or fistulas. Increased risk of cancer. Eyes may be affected: acute and chronic iridocyclitis, episcleritis, keratopathy, panuveitis, vasculitis.

Curschmann-Steinert mucular dystrophy (progressive myotonic m.d.): AD (19q13.2–q13.3). Onset in adolescence or adulthood. Affects muscles of face (myotonic facies), chewing, swallowing, neck, distal arms and legs. Myotonic cataract very common, almost always bilateral; at first punctate, whitish and colored, shiny clouding, especially in the middle cortical layers ('Christmas tree decoration'), progressive clouding, especially in the posterior lens cortex. Frequently ptosis. Rarely fixed pupils. The severe congenital form, with marked 'floppy infant' syndrome, is always inherited from the mother.

Cystinosis: AR. Metabolic disease. Increased deposition of cystine crystals in the cornea, sometimes also in conjunctiva and iris. A separate form of renal involvement in children and in adults is distinguished. Retinal involvement is possible in the renal and intermediate forms.

de Lange syndrome: Cornelia de Lange syndrome.

Demodex blepharitis: Demodex is the most common ectoparasite in humans. It can be demonstrated in many cases of chronic blepharitis by examining epilated eyelashes under the microscope. Antibiotics not sufficient to eliminate the demodex blepharitis and promotes long-term resistance of the associated flora. 2% mercury ointment and lindane are effective, but are difficult to apply and toxic.

Devic's syndrome (optic neuromyelitis): Variant of multiple sclerosis with bilateral involvement of the optic nerve in close temporal relationship to transverse myelitis.

Diabetes mellitus: Possible form of eye involvement: a) diabetic retinopathy; b) diabetic papillopathy (moderate loss of vision with papilledema, which usually disappears spontaneously within 6 months; usually in type I diabetics (children and young adults); c) diabetic pupillopathy; d) isolated outer oculomotor paresis (pupils react normally; frequently severe retro-orbital pain); e) neuroparalytic keratitis (loss of sensation).

Dorsolateral medulla oblongata syndrome: Wallenberg's syndrome.

Down's syndrome (trisomy 21, mongolism): Cardinal symptoms: hypotonia, round and flat face, mongoloid slant of palpebral fissures, small and low-set ears, short neck, four-finger crease. Possible eye changes: Brushfield's white spots on iris, epicanthal folds, congenital and juvenile cataract, myopia, iris hypoplasia, keratoconus, blepharitis, nystagmus and glaucoma.

Duane's syndrome (retraction syndrome of Duane-Stilling–Türk): Congenital VIth cranial nerve defect. Lateral rectus muscle is instead variably innervated by neurones of the IIIrd nerve, which are normally assigned to the medial rectus muscle. Cardinal symptoms: 1) impairment of abduction and adduction; 2) retraction of globe on intended adduction, with secondary narrowing of palpebral fissure. Despite considerable impairment of motility, on looking straight ahead there is usually only slight squinting and often binocular vision with slight head turning: type I: slight abduction, adduction greatly impaired (most common); type II: slight abduction, adduction greatly impaired; type III: markedly impaired abduction and adduction (up-shoot phenomenon).

Dystrophic myotonia: Curschmann-Steinert muscular dystrophy.

Eales' disease: Recurrent vitreous bleedings due to changes in the peripheral retina. Findings similar to those in sickle-cell retinopathy. Contrary to findings in, also very rare, primary periphlebitis; there are no inflammatory cells in the vitreous.

Edward's syndrome (trisomy 18): Microcephaly, hypertelorism, narrow palpebral fissure, small chin, cardiac defect, extreme mental retardation. Possible eye involvements: epicanthus, belpharophimosis, microphthalmos, dysgenetic glaucome, retinal dysplasia.

Ehlers-Danlos syndrome: A group of diseases in which connective-tissue dysplasias (abnormalities of collagen metabolism) are prominent: hyperflexible joints, lax skin, skin easily damaged and slow healing, angioid streaks (breaks in Bruch's membrane). Blue sclera, especially in type VI (ocular type), microcornea.

Eosinophilic granuloma: Histiocytosis X.

Epidermolysis, acute toxic (acute toxic necrolysis; Lyell's syndrome; syndrome of the scalded skin): acute general decline (necrotization and peeling as well as vesicles of nearly the whole upper layer of the skin without significant inflammatory reaction). Clinically similar to scalded skin and typically with positive Nikolsky phenomenon. Usually severe general reaction with splenomegaly, adrenocortical necrosis, bronchopneumonia, toxic nephrosis, cardiac hypertrophy. High death rate. Two etiological forms are distinguished: 1) caused by drug(s) (toxic epidermal necrolysis) – toxic-allergic reaction; 2) caused by staphylococcal toxin largely affects newborns and infants, young children and immunologically compromised adults.

Erythema exudativum multiforme: Acute-onset allergic dermatitis (most often postherpetic, but also after drugs). The most severe form is rare and associated with serious systemic symptoms; also called Stevens-Johnson syndrome. Conjunctivitis of varying degree in 90% of cases, sometimes with vesicles and symblepharon. If significant mucosal changes in eyes and mouth the condition is also called Fuchs' or Fiessinger-Rendu syndrome.

Essential iris atrophy: Iridocorneal endothelial dystrophy.

Fabry's disease: Glycosphingolipidosis. Deficiency of α–galactosidase. XR. Involvement of visceral organs, nervous sytem (mainly sensory neuropathy) and especially also blood vessels (aneurysmal vascular dilatations). Deposition of galactosylglucosylceramide. Cornea verticillata or radial pinnated subcapsular clouding of the lens.

Familial adenomatous polyposis: Polyposis coli.

Familial exudative vitreoretinopathy (Criswick-Schepens): AD. Exudation from abnormal retinal vessels in the temporal periphery which have become more permeable; always bilateral. The retina at the posterior pole is displaced temporally, similar to retinopathy of the premature (macular ectopia). In ca. 20% of cases the condition is progressive (pseudouveitis, retinal detachment, recurrent vitreous bleeding, proliferative vitreoretinopathy.

Felty's syndrome: Special form of rheumatoid arthritis. Splenomegaly, granulocytopenia, prone to infection.

Fibrosis syndrome: AD. Congenital, often bilateral, fibrosis of the outer eye muscles of differing degrees. Fixation of the eyes on direct gaze, ptosis or pseudoptosis (as a result of impaired elevation), paradoxical eye movements.

Fiessinger-Rendy syndrome: Erythema exudativum multiforme.

Fisher syndrome: Triad of external ophthalmoplegia, ataxia and areflexia of unknown cause. More common in juveniles.

Fissura orbitalis superior syndrome: see orbital fissure, superior.

Floppy eyelid syndrome: Disease, of unknown cause, in which there is a slack upper lid with definitely diminished consistency of the tarsus. The upper lid spontaneously everts at night during sleep. This causes conjunctival irritation resulting in chronic upper tarsal papillary conjunctivitis.

Forsius-Erikkson syndrome: Aland island eye disease.

Foster-Kennedy syndrome: Kennedy's syndrome.

Foville's syndrome (ventrocaudal brain-stem syndrome): Gaze or abducens paresis (abducens nucleus or root), sometimes ipsilateral facial paresis, as well as contralateral hemiparesis and sometimes hemianesthesia.

Franceschetti's syndrome (mandibulofacial dyostosis; Treacher-Collins syndrome: Dysmorphic syndrome with characteristic features: so-called bird's face, antimongoloid palpebral fissures, kink and colobomas of outer third of lower eyelids.

Friedreich's ataxia: AR (9p22-CEN). Progressive spinocerebellar degeneration with intial manifestation around puberty. Degeneration of mainly the posterior column of the spinal cord and of the spinocerebellar tracts together with damage to the pyramidal tract. As a result, the patient will be wheel-chair bound after an average of 15 years. The cardinal clinical symptoms are ataxia, areflexia and abnormal posterior column sensory function (loss of vibratory sense, 2-point discrimination and proprioception), especially in the feet, as well as cardiomyopathy. Gaze nystagmus, especially after saccadic eye movement, reduced fixation suppression of the vestibulo-ocular reflex and decreased optokinetic nystagmus as signs of cerebellar degeneration in the later course of the disease. Mild to moderate optic nerve atrophy in nearly half of the affected patients.

Fuchs' heterochromic cyclitis: Disease characterized by mild iridocyclitis, heterochromia of the iris, cataracts and occasionally glaucoma. As a rule it occurs unilaterally. Posterior synechiae rule out heterochromic cyclitis. Only minimal intraocular irritation (cell count +, Tyndall +. The condition is usually recognized in the 3rd to 4th decade because of the increasing cataract formation. Neovascularization on the iris and chamber angle is rare.

Fuchs' syndrome: I. Erythema exudativum multiforme. II. Corneal endothelial dystrophy.

Fundus albipunctatus: Congenital stationary night-blindness (CSNB).

Galactosemia: AR. Most common form is deficiency of galactose-1-phosphate-uridyl-transferase. Milk intolerance. Cataracts in the form of punctate or dust–like lamellar clouding in the fetal lens nucleus.

Gardner's syndrome: Polyposis coli (familial adenomatous p.); in addition, epidermoid cysts and multiple osteomas.

Gaucher's disease: AR. Lipid storage disease. Deficiency of glucocerebrosidase. Subdivided into visceral, neuropathic and subacute forms.

Glaucomatocyclytic crisis: Posner-Schlossmann syndrome.

GM_2-gangliosidosis type I: Tay-Sachs disease.

Goldenhar's syndrome (oculo-auriculovertebral dysplasia): Group of unilateral malformations. Pre-auricular ear tags, coloboma, dermoid, hemiatrophy of ipsilateral half of the face.

Goldmann-Favre syndrome: AR. It is characterized by night blindness, concentric reduction of the visual fields and impaired vision. There is a cystoid change in the macula, peripheral retinochoroid dystrophy and, in some cases, peripheral retinoschisis. An ERG is essential for differentiating this syndrome from X-chromosomal retinoschisis or retinitis pigmentosa by demonstrating a lengthened B-wave peak time and a similar tracing in both dark and light adaptation. The 'enhanced S cone syndrome' is a mild form of it.

Gorlin-Goltz syndrome (nevoid basiloma syndrome): AD. Multiple basilomas in the face, trunk, neck, arms; maxillary cysts; skeletal abnormalities, neurological abnormalities such as cerebellar medulloblastoma and calcification of the dura. Ovarian cysts, testicular disease. Hypertelorism and dystopia canthorum, strabismus, glaucoma, congenital cataract, colboma. Usually becomes manifest around puberty. In rare cases an invasive basiloma may require removal of the eye.

Gradenigo's syndrome (petrosum syndrome): Ipsilateral abducens paresis with neuralgia primarily in the area supplied by the ophthalmic nerve (first branch of the trigeminal nerve), later may also involve the region of the maxilla and mandibulum. Most cases caused by otitis and mastoiditis.

Gregg's triad: Rubella embryopathy.

Gruber-Meckel   syndrome   (dysencephalia   splanchnocystica): AR. Encephalocele, cystic renal changes, polydactylism. Occasionally microphthalmos, coloboma, cataract.

Haltia's disease: Neuronal ceroid lipofuscinosis.

Hand-Schüller-Christian disease: Histiocytosis X.

Harada's syndrome: Vogt-Koynagi-Harada syndrome.

Heerfordt's syndrome: Sarcoidosis.

Hermansky-Pudlak syndrome: AR. Oculocutaneous albinism with variable phenotype within affected families. Further symptoms: hemorrhagic diathesis (platelet defect), pigmented reticular cells and abnormal ceroid deposition, especially in the lung, heart and kidneys. The morbidity and mortality of the disease is determined by the state of the organs affected.

Hertwig-Magendie squint (skew deviation): Vertical squint possibly due to supranuclear lesion. Site of lesion: otoliths (peripheral); entire brainstem, from diencephalon to medulla (central). If caudal brainstem is affected, ipsilateral eye is lower. Alternating skew deviation if lesion in midbrain tegmentum, cervicomedullary transition or cerebellar.

Heterochromic cyclitis: Fuchs' heterochromic cyclitis.

Hippel-Lindau syndrome: AD inherited phacomatosis. Prevalence 1 : 40 000; defective gene on chromosome 3p25–26 (probably suppressor gene). Main signs: a) hemangioblastomas in cerebellum and other CNS regions (so-called Lindau tumors) as well as uni- or bilateral retinal angiomatosis; b) clear-cell renal carcinoma; c) pheochromocytoma; and d) polycystic organs (liver, pancreas, kidney, epididymis). Minimal criteria for diagnosis: retinal angiomatosis or CNS hemangioblastoma and, in patient or first-degree relative, one of the above main manfestations.

Histiocytosis X: Generic term for the reticuloendothelioses: **Abt-Letterer-Siwe** (only in children, possibly orbital tumors); **Hand-Christian-Schüller** (defects of the skull bones, exphthalmos, diabetes insipidus); **eosinophilic granuloma** (unifocal osteolysis).

Histoplasmosis syndrome (so-called ocular histoplasmosis syndrome; idiopathic subretinal neovascularization): A fungal infection endemic in North America. Ocular histoplasmosis cannot be distinguished clinically from idiopathic posterior subretinal neovascularization. Through the ophthalmoscope: 'histospots' (multifocal, atrophic changes in the choroid), parafoveal subretinal neovascularization and a conus with internal pigment ring.

Homocystinuria: Heterogeneous picture with variable response to treatment with vitamin B_6. Usually starts in first decade with lenticular ectopia (mostly towards nose and downward), occasionally cataract, glaucoma, retinal degeneration, myopia and astigmatism, thrombotic vascular occlusions.

Horner's syndrome: Miosis, ptosis and apparent enophthalmos (raised position of lower lid);

– **postganglionic:** in cluster headache, tumor or fracture at base of skull, metastases and inflammation of the cervical lymph nodes;

– **preganglionic:** in tumors of the neck and cervicothoracic regions (shoulder-arm pain associated with Horner's s. points to bronchogenic carcinoma: Pancoast tumor). Neoplasia more common than with postganglionic Horner's s.

– **central:** In brainstem infarction (Wallenberg's syndrome); cortical lesion.

Horton's disease: Temporal arteritis.
Hunter's disease: Mucopolysaccharidosis.
Hurler's diasease: Mucopolysaccharidosis.
Hutchinson's triad: 1) Hutchinson teeth (barrel-shaped malformation, particularly of the upper incisors); 2) parenchymatous keratitis; 3) inner-ear deafness in congenital syphilis.
Hydrocephalus: Enlargement of the cerebrospinal fluid (CSF) spaces of various causes. **Internal h.:** enlarged ventricles; **external h.:** enlargement of the subarachnoid space; **obstructive h.:** obstruction of CSF flow; **hypersecreting h.:** increased CSF production; **nonabsorptive h.:** decreased CSF absorption; danger of optic nerve damage. In older children and adults the most important symptoms are headache, double vision (eye muscle paresis), and papilledema.
Incontinentia pigmenti Bloch Sulzberger: X-chromosome inherited skin anomaly, lethal in males. At first, at birth or soon after, vesicular then verrucous efflorescences, later pigmentation. Bilateral ocular involvement in 30%: myopia, strabismus, microphthalmos, corneal and lenticular opacification.
Internuclear ophthalmoplegia (INO): Slow or impaired adduction of one eye with nystagmus of the abducted other eye (dissociated nystagmus); this nystagmus opposite the lesion is not always present. Proof of INO: one eye cannot be adducted when changing direction of gaze but only by near-vision convergence. If unilateral INO in elderly patient: usual cause is ischemia (brainstem). Bilateral INO in young patient: usually multiple sclerosis.
Iridocorneoendothelial (ICE) dystrophy: Abnormally increased formation of Descemet's membrane by endothelium; deposits in iridocorneal angle and on iris; iris atrophy, almost always unilateral. 3 classical pictures are distinguished: **(1) essential iris atrophy** (iris stroma atrophy, anterior synechiae, pupillary distortion); **(2) iris nevus syndrome (Cogan-Reese)** (anterior surface of iris has whitish discolorations, in between nodules of normal dark iris tissue); **(3) Chandler's syndrome** (early endothelial decompensation.
Iridotrabeculocorneal dysgenesis (anterior chamber cleavage syndrome, mesodermal or mesenchymal dysgenesis): AD developmental abnormality. Iris stroma hypoplasia and synechiae between iris and cornea. **Posterior embryotoxon** (prominent Schwalbe's line). **Axenfeld's anomaly** (prominent Schwalbe's line and iris processes). **Posterior circumscribed keratoconus** (thinning of the posterior stroma with indentation of the intact endothelium and of Descemet's membrane). **Peters' anomaly** (iris connected to posterior surface of central cornea). **Rieger's syndrome** (iridocorneal adhesions, additionally maxillary hypoplasia and tooth anomalies). Glaucoma in ca. 50% of cases.
Iris nevus syndrome (Cogan-Reese): Iridocorneoendothelial dystrophy.
Jansky-Bielschowsky disease: Late juvenile form of neuronal ceroid lipofuscinosis.
Kartagener syndrome: Primary ciliary dyskinesia syndrome. Genetically determined disorder of mucociliary apparatus with impaired secretion. Bronchiectasis and chronic rhinosinusitis, sperm immobility. Situs inversus. Possible ophthalmological malformations.
Kearns-Sayre syndrome: External ophthlmoplegia with bilateral ptosis, dystrophy of retinal pigment epithelium, cardiac conduction abnormalities, increased CSF protein. Manifests itself before aged 20 years. Caused by mito-

chondrial abnormality (maternal inheritance). Special form of chronic progressive external ophthalmoplegia (CPEO).

Kennedy's syndrome: Combination of unilateral ophthalmoplegia with contralateral papilledema. Most common cause is slowly enlarging space-occupying lesion near the optic canal, resulting at first in homolateral optic nerve atrophy and later in an increase in CSF pressure.

Cerebellopontine syndrome: Facial paresis, trigeminal involvement, hearing impairment, possibly tinnitus, suggestive cerebellar and contralacteral pyramidal signs.

Laurence-Moon syndrome: Bardet-Biedl syndrome.

Leber's optic atrophy, hereditary Leber's optic neuropathy (LHON): Mitochondrial abnormality with maternal inheritance, affecting males five times more often than females. At the onset, unilateral then (after an interval of several weeks to months) bilateral acute or subacute marked loss of vision in otherwise completely healthy persons. Typical age at onset between 18 and 30 years, but it can manifest itself at any age. There is a central or cecocentral scotoma and marked dyschromatopsia. Fundoscopically there is a triad of indistinct disc margin, peripapillary microangiopathy and no leakage of fluorescence from the teleangiectatic vessels. Within weeks or months the vascular changes regress and subsequently the disc becomes pale. Final visual acuity will be 0.1 or worse. The diagnosis is confirmed by molecular genetic tests.

Leber's congenital amaurosis (LCA): Heterogeneous group of tapetoretinal dystrophies which manifest themselves from birth or in the first 8 years of life in the form of marked visual disturbances, even blindness, with reduced or extinguished ERG responses. Group 1: congenital blindness, extinguished ERG responses and hyperopia. Group 2: Additional systemic diseases. Groups 3 and 4: Can be termed as juvenile (manifestation by the second year) or as early adult retinitis pigmentosa (manifestation by the eighth year).

Leigh's syndrome: Subacute necrotizing encephalopathy caused by a congenital mitochondrial abnormality in the upper brainstem. Muscular hypotonia. Cranial nerves affected. Death between 1st and 5th year of life.

LEOPARD syndrome (cardiocutaneous syndrome): AD. Combination of changes with characteristic skin condition. The skin seems to be freckled, due to numerous dark lentigines. The term is an acronym made up of the different characteristics of the disease: **l**entigines (>80%), **e**lectrocardiographic abnormalities (<80%), **o**cular hypertelorism (c. 75%), **p**ulmonary valve stenosis (<80%), **a**bnormal genitals (in males), **r**etarded growth (<80%), **d**eafness (c. 15%).

Leptospirosis: Weil's disease.

Lipoid proteinosis Urbach-Wiethe (cutaneous and mucosal hyalinosis): Rare systemic disease. can lead to pearl necklace-like changes at the lid edges and secondarily to keratoconjunctivitis sicca. Exceptionally it may have intraocular changes in the form of drusen-like fundal deposits.

Little's syndrome (infantile cerebral palsy): Generic term for final stages of intrauterine or perinatal cerebral damage.

Löfgren's syndrome: Sarcoidosis.

Louis Bar's syndrome (ataxia teleangiectatica): AR. Inherited disease with increased chromosomal instability (fragile chromosome sites). Progressive cerebral ataxia. Thymus dysplasia with lymphopenia and IgA deficiency, combined with oculocutaneous teleangiectasia. Diagnosis occasionally possible because of conjunctival changes.

Lowe's syndrome (oculocerebrorenal s.): sex-liked disease with generalized hyperaminoacidosis resulting from renal tubular insufficiency. Physical and mental retardation. Cataract in almost all cases, manifesting itself between birth and 6 months, and glaucoma, in about 2/3 of patients, usually bilateral. Other ocular findings: microphthalmos, strabismus. nystagmus, miosis and iris atrophy. Female carriers can be detected by having cortical lenticular opacities and through genetic tests.

Lyell's syndrome: Epidermolysis, acute toxic.

Manibulopalpebral synkinesia (Marcus Gunn phenomenon): Elevation of ptotic lid on opening mouth and moving lower jaw to other side. Caused by congenital coupling of innervation between the levator palpebrae muscle and the ipsilateral pterygoid muscle (pulls the mandible forward on opening of the mouth).

Marcus Gunn syndrome: Mandibulopalpebral synkinesia.

Marfan's syndrome (arachnodactyly): AD-inherited gene coding the synthesis of fibrillin, the main component of microfibrils which are found in elastic fibers but also play an important part in anchoring the collagen in connective tissue. Strict diagnostic criteria: lens luxation (usually upward and temporal). Aortic dilatation, severe kyphoscoliosis, ventral thoracic deformity. Other criteria: myopia, mitral valve prolapse, tall stature, joint hyperflexibility, arachnodactyly. 90% of patients have one or more cardiovascular abnormalities which are responsible for limited life expectancy without treatment.

Marin-Amat syndrome: Increase in unilateral, moderate ptosis on opening the mouth and sideward movement of the jaw. Probably due to co-innervation of orbicularis oculi and chewing muscles.

Maroteaux-Lamy disease: Mucopolysaccharidosis.

Marshall's syndrome: Myopia, vitreoretinal degeneration, short stature and typical facial changes (saddle nose). Outward appearance Stickler's syndrome.

Meige's syndrome: Essential blepharospasm combined with oromandibular dystonia.

Melkersson-Rosenthal syndrome: Recurrent granulomatosis of unknown cause with recurrent swelling of the lips (cheilitis granulomatosa), facial paresis, scrotal tongue.

Mikulicz's syndrome: Sarcoidosis.

Millard-Gubler syndrome (alternating facial hemiplegia): Facial paresis (2. motor neurone of facial nerve) on the side of the lesion, contralateral motor hemiparesis (pyramidal tract in the pontine bulb). Sometimes also ipsilateral abduction paresis.

Mixed-solution syndrome: Toxic corneal lesion after changing cleansing fluid for contact lenses (which contain quaternary ammonium base and chlorhexidine gluconate).

Möbius's syndrome (congenital oculofacial paresis): Bilateral facial paresis and abnormal eye movements, usually abduction paresis and/or horizontal gaze paresis. Intact vertical movement and Bell's phenomenon. Aplasia or hypoplasia of VI. and VII. nerves.

Morning glory syndrome (disc dysplasia): Papillary dysplasia.

Morquio's disease: Mucopolysaccharidosis.

Mucopolysaccharidoses: AR. Storage diseases whose common abnormality is a defect in the lysosomal breakdown of complex carbohydrates, the mucopolysaccharides. **Type I (Hurler's disease):** coarse facial features, macroglossia, thickened skin, corneal opacity, rarely glaucoma.

Hepatosplenomegaly, joint contractures and disproportionate small stature. Mild forms with nearly normal life expectancy are called **Schele's disease**. X-chromosomal inheritance is found in **type II (Hunter's disease)**, in which there is usually no corneal opacification. **Type III (Sanfilippo's disease)** is characterized by rapid cerebral degeneration with usually only minor dysmorphic signs. In **Type IV (Morquio's disease)** the skeletal abnormalities predominate. Patients with **type V (Maroteaux-Lamy disease)** is outwardly like Hurler's disease (such as corneal opacity, rarely glaucoma), but they have normal intelligence.

Myasthenia gravis: Functional abnormality at the neuromuscular junction due to blockage of the acetylcholine receptors by autoreactive antibodies of the IgG type (autoimmune disease). Ocular symptoms are the most frequent initial feature, but in most cases there follows secondary generalization of symptoms. Ocular myasthenia can in principle imitate all other patterns of motor disorders. To be included in the differential diagnosis if paresis without ocular sings and without pupillary involvement. Generalized forms: young adult form (predominantly females) with lymphofollicular thymus hyperplasia; senile form: equally frequent in males and females. Congenital forms are genetically, not immunologically, determined.

Neurofibromatosis (Recklinghausen's disease): AD. Developmental abnormality affecting skin, nervous system and internal organs. Neurofibromas of the peripheral, central and autonomic nervous systems, skin pigmentations. 50% of children with an optic glioma (astrocytoma of the optic fascicle) have the disease. Type 1 is the most common form (defect of the NF-1 tumor suppressor gene, located on chromosome 22q11; type 2 ic characterized by bilateral acoustic neuromas (defect of NH-2 gene on 22q11).

Neurocutaneous syndrome (phacomatoses): neurofibromatosis, tuberous sclerosis, Struge-Weber syndrome, Hipple-Lindau disease.

Neuronal ceroid lipofuscinoses (NCL, Batten's disease): AR. Group of neurodegenerative diseases of childhood generally characterized by a syndrome of 'amaurotic dementia' with loss of vision, loss of psychomotor functions and epilepsy. **Juvenile form (Spielmeyer-Vogt) disease,** the most common form (incidence 0.7 : 100 000), develops in at first completely healthy children who, between 4 and 7 years of age, begin to loose their sight, with blindness on average when aged 10; progressive retinal degeneration with abnormal ERG. **Late infantile form (Jansky-Bielschowsky disease):** hardly less common. It begins in children aged between 2 and 4 years with severe drug–resistant epilepsy; despite progressive retinal degeneration vision remains at first relatively good. Very rare are the **infantile or Finnish form (Santavuori-Haltia disease),** the **adult form (Kufs' disease),** and the **Finnish variant of late-infantile NCL.** In all forms the diagnosis is confirmed by electronmicroscopic demonstration of disease-specific lipopigments, e.g. in circulating lymphocytes.

Niemann-Pick disease: AR. Sphingomyelin lipidosis. Lack of lysosomal sphingomyelinase. As a result the cells of the macrophage system as well as the glial and ganglion cells store sphingomyelins (foam cells). In addition to symptoms as in Tay-Sachs disease (such as cherry-red spots), there is also marked hepatosplenomegaly.

Norrie's disease: Leukocoria due to dysplastic retina, bilateral hearing impairment (in 1/3 of cases), mental retardation (2/3 of cases). X-chromosomal recessive inheritance, i.e. only boys are affected.

Nothnagel's syndrome: III. nerve paresis with ipsilateral cerebellar ataxia.

Nucleus ruber syndrome: Benedikt's syndrome.

Oblique superior click syndrome: Intermittent impairment of lifting eyes in adduction. When doing this the patient sometimes feels a painful click caused by thickened tendon in the trochlear region.

Oblique superior myokymia: Superior oblique myokomia.

Oguchi's disease: Congenital stationary night blindness (CSNB).

Oculomotor apraxia (Cogan's syndrome): Inability to initiate focused gaze; congenital or acquired (Huntington's chorea, brainstem tumor, etc.).

Oculopharyngeal muscular dystrophy: AD. Ptosis and dysphagia, rarely ophthalmoplegia. Most common among French Canadians.

Oculocerebrorenal syndrome: Lowe's syndrome.

Ophthalmoplegia: Chronic progressive external ophthalmoplegia.

Opsoclonus: Salvo-like, rapid, conjugated, predominantly horizontal saccades of differing amplitudes without fixed intervals (6–12 Hz), spontaneous or induced by eye movements. Frequently additional cerebellar symptoms such as trunk ataxia, dysarthria, limb clonus. Occurs in encephalitis, paraneoplastic syndrome (neuroblastoma in children), bleeding, infarcts, intoxication.

Optic atrophy, juvenile: autosomal dominant optic nerve atrophy.

Orbital fissure, superior: Complete or partial combination of paresis of the abducens, oculomotor, trochlear, frontal, lacrimal and nasociliary nerves. In some cases retro-orbital pain and exophthalmos.

Osteogenesis imperfecta: Group of diseases characterized by brittle bones. Caused by gene defects in collagen I and III. Blue sclerae, especially in type II.

Parinaud's syndrome: Supranuclear disorder of eye movements. Complete paralysis of vertical gaze (most frequent form) or isolated paralysis of upward and downward gaze. Upper lid retraction and convergent nystagmus on attempting to look up. Usually tonic pupils. In classical form, unable to move eyes upward, fixed pupils, sometimes retraction nystagmus.

Patau's syndrome (trisomy 13–15): Cardinal symptoms: cleft lips, maxilla and palate. Microphthalmia, hexadactyly, agyria (no cortical gyri), lissencephaly (only slight divisions of the cerebral cortex into gyri). Other possible ocular findings: coloboma, retinal dysplasia, congenital cataract, lens dislocation, dysembryogenesis of the iridocorneal angle.

Peters' anomaly: Iridotrabeculocorneal dysgenesis.

Peutz-Jeghers syndrome: AD. Lentigopolyposis. Mucocutaneous mid-brown pigmented spots, particularly of lip and buccal mucosa. Gastrointestinal, especially small-intestinal, polyposis. High risk of colorectal cancer.

Pfundler–Hurler disease: Mucopolysaccharidoses.

Phacomatosis-associated tumors: AD-inherited syndrome of variable penetrance, with tumors or tumor-like malformations of the nervous system, skin and internal organs. Most important tumors are: neurofibroma, tuberous sclerosis, Hippel-Lindau syndrome, Sturge-Weber syndrome.

Phytanic acid lipidosis: Refsum's disease.

Pierre Robin's syndrome: Early fetal malformations in the region of mouth and tongue. Micrognathia, glossoptosis, cleft palate. Occasionally progressive cataract, microphthalmia, glaucoma.

Pigment dispersion syndrome: Triad of 1) radial defect of iris pigment layer (no stromal defect); 2) pigment deposition on corneal epithelium, typically as vertical Krukenberg spindle; circular pigmentation of trabecular network, of unknown cause; rubbing of iris pigment layer against the zonular fibers when anterior chamber is deep (moderate myopia); glaucoma in 10%; intraocular pressure increase often improves with advancing age. Usually bilateral, but asymmetrical.

Polyposis of colon; familial adenomatous polyposis (FAP): True precancerous lesion. Hundreds of colorectal polyps. First manifestation usually in second decade. In c. 85% of those affected there are areas of congenital hypertrophy of the retinal pigment epithelium (CHRPE). When a person at risk has CHRPE, it suggests FAP-gene carrier status. Negative fundus findings can be interpreted as indicating lower risk only if other members of the patients's family with FAP also have CHRPE.

Posner-Schlossmann   syndrome   (glaucomatocyclitic   crisis): Intermittent, often drastic, rise in inner eye pressure, persisting for days or even weeks, with few symptoms. Usually no loss of function, but wide-angle glaucoma may develop. Steroids and anti-glaucoma drugs usually effective in inhibiting chamber water production (carbonic anhydrase inhibitors, beta blockers). Possible immunological cause.

Prader-Willi syndrome: Deletion of 15q11. Retardation syndrome with characteristic features. Narrow forehead, sunken temporal region, upward slanting lid axes. Obesity, marked muscular hypotonia. Oculocutaneous albinism and congenital uveal ectropion, which is associated with open-angle glaucoma.

Progressive myotonic muscular dystrophy: Curschmann-Steinert disease.

Putscher's disease (traumatic angiopathy): Retinal vasculitis after ordinary accident without direct damage to eyes, caused by microemboli (shock syndrome). Rare occurrence in nontraumatic pancreatitis.

Raeder's syndrome: (Peripheral) Horner's syndrome and headache in area innervated by 1. trigeminal branch. Closely related to cluster headache.

Refsum's disease (phytanic acid lipidosis, heredopathia atactica polyneuritiformis): AR defect of phytanic acid-α-hydroxylase: phytanic acid accumulates in tissues. Result of phytanic acid incorporation in the myelin is ganglion cell necrosis and myelin sheath destruction with corresponding clinical symptoms. Associated symptoms and findings may anticipate by years the neurological changes. The latter are: painful paresthesias, swollen peripheral nerve endings, muscle weakness of distal limbs, anosmia, miosis, inner-ear deafness, dysphagia, cerebellar signs and disorders of cardiac conduction system. Occasionally, ichthyosis, rarely posterior subcapsular lenticular clouding. Progression of the disease can be arrested with low phytanic acid diet and monitoring serum phytanic acid levels.

Reiter's syndrome (urethro-oculosynovial s.): Occurs as part of an intestinal or genitourinary infection, especially in persons with HLA-B27 expression (2/3 of cases). Symptoms: a) (poly)arthritis of the large joints and the sacroiliac joints (nearly almost: knee), similar to Bechterew's disease; b) urethritis (nongonococcal, possibly nonmicrobial); c) ocular involvement: mucopurulent and even follicular conjunctivitis (in 60% of cases), variable iridocyclitis (in 10–20%); rarely keratitis and episcleritis. Usually affects young men (M : F-9 : 1).

Retinitis pigmentosa (RP): Group of hereditary diseases, characterized by night-blindness and reduction of visual field. Forms: **classical RP:** triad of pigment deposition, attenuated retinal arteries and waxy pallor of optic disc. When RP is suspected, absence of myopia speaks against the diagnosis. Modes of inheritance: 1) AR (ca. 50%, early onset); 2) AD (ca. 20%, later onset, relatively benign). 3) X-linked R, rare, similar to (1). **Atypical RP:** no pigmentation, retinitis punctata albescens (multiple white atrophic spots), segmental RP (most frequent in the inferior retinal quadrant, AD). **Phenotypes:** acquired diseases can have symptoms and findings similar to RP. To be excluded are syphilis, congenital rubella, chronic recurrent posterior uvcitis, vitamin A deficicncy, as well as side effects of drugs, e.g. chlorpromazine, thiodiazine and chloroquine.

RP-associated syndromes: Numerous syndromes may be associated with RP. Frequently it is a cone-rod dystrophy. Among such diseases are: mucopolysaccharidoses, peroxysomal and mitochondrial disorders (Kearns-Sayre s.), as well as others, some of them treatable (Usher's s., Bardett-Biedl s., Bassen-Kornzweig s., Refsum's disease, atrophia gyrata).

Richner–Harnhart syndrome: Herpes-like corneal dystrophy, palmoplantar keratoses, later oligophrenia. Metabolic disorder with tyrosinemia.

Rieger's syndrome: Iris hypoplasia, chamber angle anomaly, posterior embryotoxon (its absence practially excludes Rieger's s.), reduced dentition and microdontia; iridotrabeculocorneal dysgenesis.

Rift valley fever: Caused by an RNA-virus of the Arbovirus genus with fever, headache, joint pains and often marked photophobia. One to three weeks after onset retinitis with vasculitis may develop. Endemic in southern Africa.

Riley-Day syndrome (hereditary sensory and autonomic neuropathy type III [HSAN III]): Disease starts at birth: Cell loss in sensory and peripheral autonomic ganglia. Nearly total analgesia, loss of thermoregulation, hyposmia, no lacrimation and secondary keratitis.

Robin's syndrome: Pierre Robin syndrome.

Rocky Mountain spotted fever: One of several, closely related, influenza-like tick-borne rickettsial diseases. Various and differing ocular involvements: conjunctivitis, subconjunctival bledings, papilledema, cotton-wool foci, retinal hemorrhages, occlusion of retinal vessels.

Ross' syndrome: Pupillotonia and fixed accomodation with abnormal sweating (segmental anhidrosis).

Rothmund's syndrome: AR. Poikiloderma with cutaneous atrophy ('marmorization') and facial teleangiectasias. Shield-shaped anterior and posterior lens capsule, manifesting itself during the 2nd to 4th year of life.

Rubella embryopathy: Gregg's triad of cataract, deafness and cardiovascular defects. Possible ophthalmological findings: microphthalmia (uni- or bilateral), congenital cataract, pseudoretinitis pigmentosa (normal ERG! No dystrophy). No progression of symptoms.

Sanfilippo's disease: Mucopolysaccharidosis.

Santavuori-Haltia disease: Neuronal ceroid lipofuscinosis.

Sarcoidosis: Systemic ganulomatosis, predominantly affecting the lungs and intrathoracic lymph nodes. Ocular involvement in about 1/3 of cases, most often chronic; granulomatous iridocyclitis (in half of those with ocular involvement), more rarely granulomas of iris and/or conjunctiva. Can imitate practically any intraocular inflammation (periphlebitis, chorioretinitis etc.). 90% of patients with ocular findings have also pulmonary involvement (chest x-ray). **Löfgren's syndrome** (acute sacrcoidosis: hilar adenopathy, erythema nodosum, arthralgias, anterior uveitis); **Heerford's syndrome** (facial paralysis, parotid swelling, uveitis, fever); **Miculicz syndrome** (swelling of tear- and salivary glands).

Scheie's disease: Mucopolysaccharidosis.

Sheehan's syndrome: Panhypopituitarism caused by extensive necroses of the maternal hypophysis after post-partum shock; may be associated with peripheral field defects.

Shy-Drager syndrome: Degenerative disease of the lateral horns of the spinal cord, the caudate nucleus and cranial nerve nuclei, with progressive failure of autonomic nervous system function. Orthostatic hypotension; parkinsonian facies, tonic pupils.

Sialidosis: Storage disease. Increased urinary concentration of oligosaccharides. Possible other abnormalities: ataxia, progressive myoclonic epilepsy, macular degeneration (cherry-red spot).

Sinus cavernosus syndrome: partial or complete combination of paresis of abducens, trochlear, frontal, lacrimal and nasociliary nerves; possibly also of the V_2 nerve; cf. carotid-cavernous sinus fistula.

Sluder syndrome: Paroxysmal unilateral conjunctival reddening, tears, rhinorrhea, periorbital neuralgia. Probable cause: neuralgia of the sphenopalatine ganglion. Cf. Charlin's syndrome.

Sorsby's (pseudoinflammatory) retinal dystrophy: AD. Progressive loss of vision in middle age due to hemorrhagic macular disease (subretinal neovascularization). Ultimately almost complete blindness.

Spielmeyer-Vogt disease: Juvenile form of neuronal ceroid lipofuscinosis.

Spondylitis, ankylosing: Bechterew's disease.

Stargardt's macular dystrophy with fundus flavimaculatus: AR, rarely AD/defect in ABCR gene on chromosome 1p. Usual onset in 1st or 2nd decade with loss of central vision without photophobia. Marked problem with color differentiation or night vision. Yellowish spots on fundus. Macula looks like 'beaten bronze'; marked variations. Ultimate visual acuity rarely worse than 0.05. Fluorescence angiography typically shows reduced background fluorescence (dark choroid), caused by deposition in the retinal pigmented. In addition there may be hyperfluorescences. Contrary to conal dystrophy, whole-field ERG is not abnormal at the beginning of the disease. In the later stages the shows a reduced rise in brightness. Fundus flavimaculatus is a special form of Stargardt' disease with bright spots at the posterior pole and the middle periphery, as well as absent or less marked central findings.

Steele-Richardson-Olszewski syndrome: Progressive gaze paralysis and parkinsonism. At first usually paralysis of downward vertical gaze, later rigid dystonia of neck and trunk, tendency to loss of balance and dysarthria.

Stevens-Johnson syndrome: Erythema exudativum multiforme.

Stickler's syndrome (hereditary progressive arthro-ophthalmopathy): AD. Multisystem disease, probably connective tissue disorder. Ocular, orofacial (mandibular hypoplasia) and musculoskeletal abnormalities. Most common ocular findings: high myopia, open-angle glaucoma, cataract and vitreoretinal degeneration (optically empty, liquified vitreous; mobile, some times dense, avascular membrane or strands; peripheral pigment deposits; equatorial degeneration). Frequently retinal detachment. Tendency to giant tears.

Still's (-Chauffard) syndrome: Form of chronic juvenile arthritis. Onset between 2nd and 4th year, with bouts of fever, polyarthralgia, myalgia, measles-like rash, hepatosplenomegaly with lymphadenopathy, polyserositis, iridocyclitis, leucocytosis and anemia in the absence of most rheumatoid factors. Most frequent combination is oligoarthritis with uveitis. Iridocyclitis with slow onset is typical. Danger of secondary glaucoma.

String sdyndrome: Ciliary neuralgia after cerclage operation.

Sturge-Weber syndrome: (1) Nevus flammeus of the face (congenital, usually in the V_2 to V_3 nerve distribution; (2) calcified angioma of the leptomeninges (leads to cerebral atrophy and epilepsy, possibly hemianopsia); (3) ocular involvement (glaucoma, usually since childhood; choroid angioma, etc.). Often not all criteria are present.

Subacute sclerosing panencephalitis (SSPE): An encephalomyelitis, caused by measles virus in the form of a slow-virus infection. In its late stage, demyelination and sclerosis. Results in myoclonias, extrapyramidal disorders, spastic paralyses, dementia. Focal retinitis, optic nerve atrophy, nystagmus and paralysis of the eye muscles.

Superior oblique myokymia: Episodic monocular microtremors resulting in diplopia and oscillopsia. Due to uncontrolled activity of single fibers of IVth cranial nerve. Occasionally may be provoked by looking downward; in this case, look for microtremors with the slit-lamp when looking ahead. Benign, often disappears spontaneously.

Superior oblique click syndrome: Oblique superior click syndrome.

Takayasu's arteritis: Arteritis that usually affects aorta of young females, aged 10–30 years (M : F = 1 : 7). Stenosis at origin of arteries arising from aorta, resulting in 'pulseless disease'. Low pressure glaucoma.

Tay-Sachs disease (GM$_2$-gangliosidosis type 1): Amaurotic idiocy = infantile GM$_2$-gangliosidosis (sphingolipidosis). Recessive inheritance. Absence of lysosomal β-N-acetylgalactosaminidase. As a result, GM$_2$-monosialoganglioside is stored in the glial and ganglion cells until these cells die. Spastic paralysis, seizures, blindness due to optic atrophy, macular 'cherry-red spots' Amaurotic dementia also caused by neuronal ceroid lipofuscinosis.

Terson's syndrome: Vitreous bleedings due to increased cerebrospinal fluid pressure. Subarachnoid hemorrhage is the most common cause. Branches of the central vein or the central vein itself are the most common source of intraocular bleeding in this syndrome.

Trochlear paralysis: IVth nerve is the thinnest of all the cranial nerves and has the longest intracranial course. It is the only nerve with a dorsal exit. Symptoms: reduced or absent downward movement in adduction; excyclotropia. Vertical deviation aggravated when head inclines towards side of paralysis (Bielschowsky's phenomenon). Often caused by head trauma.

Tolosa-Hunt syndrome: Special form of orbital pseudotumor with involvement of the cavernous sinus. Unilateral pain behind the eye with ipsilateral paralysis of IIIrd nerve (most often) and/or IVth and VIth. Sensory disorder in the 1st trigeminal branch, mild protrusion of eye. No marked signs of congestion in the eye. Other causes must be excluded (e.g. carotid-cavernous sinus fistula). Unknown etiology. Nonspecific granulomatous inflammation may be found. If patients do not respond to cortisone, another diagnosis is probable.

Trisomy: Trisomy 21 Down's syndrome; trisomy 13 Pätau's syndrome; trisomy 18 Edwards' syndrome.

Tuberous sclerosis (Bourneville-Pringle disease): AD. High penetrance. Defective gene locus on chromosome 9q. New mutations occur in ca. 50% of cases. Multiple mulberry–like astrocytic hamartomas of the retina, cerebral sclerosis, facial angiofibromas. Seizures from childhood in most cases.

Uhthoff's sign: Increased dysfunction in neuritis of the optic nerve resulting from physical exertion or an increase in body temperature.

Usher's syndrome: Retinitis pigmentosa (RP) with inner-ear deafness. 15 to 20% of all patients with RP and 50% of those with deafness and blindness have Usher's syndrome. RP is associated with congenital sensorimotor deafness (Usher I) or with stationary (Usher II) or progressive (Usher III) high-pitch hearing impairment. Usher I is associated with impaired vestibular function and nonprogressive ataxia. Signs of RP appear in the first to second (Usher I) or second to third (Usher II, III) decades. Usually AR inheritance. Cf. RP-associated syndromes.

Uveal effusion syndrome: Obstruction to drainage in the region of the vortex veins if they are aplastic or hypoplastic. Nanophthalmos, posterior scleritis or as postoperative complication, resulting in partial or circular choroidal detachment (uveal effusion).

Vogt-Koyanagi-Harada syndrome (uveoencephalitis): Autoimmune disease with panuveitis, frequent in Asia (Japan). Division into Vogt-Koyanaga syndrome (predominantly anterior uveitis) and Harada'a syndrome (predominantly posterior uveitis with serous retinal detachment) is clinically not important, because there are numerous transitional forms. V-K-H s. can be assumed when there are symptoms from at least two of the following three groups: skin changes (alopecia, vitiligo, poliosis); neurological abnormalities (headache, stiff neck, encephalopathy, hearing disorders, increased cell count in cerebrospinal fluid); uveitis.

von Hippel-Lindau syndrome: Hippel-Lindau syndrome.

Waardenburg's syndrome: AR with differing expressivity. Characteristic features are dystopia canthorum (medial canthi displaced laterally), blepharophimosis, broad nasal root, fused eyebrows. Heterochromia of the iris, deafness, white frontal hair curl. Most important symptom is the usually severe inner ear deafness (in 20%). Open angle glaucoma is uncommon, although it was present in the cases originally described by Waardenburg.

Wagner's disease: AD vitreoretinal degeneration with onset usually around 20 years of age. Optically empty vitreous with a few strands; markedly pigmented equatorial radial degeneration along the retinal vessels. Myopia, early cataract formation, high risk of complicated retinal detachment. Occurs in isolation or associated with bone dysplasia syndromes.

WAGR syndrome: Association of Wilms' tumor (W), aniridia (A); genital abnormality (G: cryptorchidism, hypospadias, hermaphroditism); and mental retardation (R). Not all symptoms may occur simultaneously. Wilms' tumor in 1/3 of patients. Variable incidence of aniridia.

Wallenberg's syndrome (dorsolateral oblongata s.): Special form of anemic cerebral infarct with usually thrombotic occlusion of the origin of the vertebral a. from the subclavian a. with extension to the main branch of the inferior posterior cerebral a. This results in infarction of the dorsolateral part of the medulla oblongata. On the side of the infarct there wil be facial paresthesias (trigeminal n.), paralysis (sometimes facial, abducens m.), soft palate paralysis and hoarseness (hypoglossal n., vagus n., glossopharyngeal n.), ataxia (spinocerebellar tract) as well as central Horner's syndrome (central sympathetic tract). On the contralateral side there will be disorders of sensation and also pyramidal signs. Occasionally ocular tilt reaction may occur (excyclotropia of the ipsilateral eye and simultaneous hypertropia of the contralateral eye).

Weber's syndrome (crus cerebri s., alternating oculomotor hemiplegia): III. nerve paralysis (nuclear or radicular lesion of the oculomotor n.) with contralateral hemiplegia, including lower half of the face (pyramidal tract with cerebral peduncle).

Wegener's granulomatosis: Necrotizing, granulomatous vasculitis. Autoimmune disease. Local or regional initial stage with antibiotic-resistant rhinitis/sinusitis (diagnosis made from mucosal biopsy and determining anticytoplasmatic antibodies). Stage of generalization with systemic vasculitis. Eye involvement varies: episcleritis or scleritis, vasculitits, diffuse choroiditis, inflammatory orbital pseudotumor.

Weil's disease (leptospirosis): Infectious disease, caused by Leptospira interrogans, with periods of fever and fever–free intervals, initial gastrointestinal symptoms. Muscle and joint pains, signs of meningeal involvement. Iridocyclitis rare in the first phase; more typical are late reactions (varying degrees of iridocyclitis) occurring after many months.

Weil-Marchesani syndrome (spherophakia-bradymorphic syndrome): AR. Microspherophakia, lens dislocation, brachydactyly, brachycephaly and growth retardation.

Werner's syndrome (progeria in adults): AR. Premature mesodermal ageing. Main symptoms: scleroderma-like skin changes; old person's thin face; vascular sclerosis; cataract, rarey corneal clouding, abnormal pigment epithelium, blue sclerae.

Wernicke's encephalopathy: Encephalopathy caused by thiamine deficiency, most common in alcoholics. In its classic form, triad of psychiatric disorder, eye symptoms (nystagmus, abducens paralysis, gaze paralysis, pupillary disorder, ptosis) and abnormal gait. Rapid regression, especially of ocular symptoms and ataxia, on early parenteral thiamine adminstration.

Whipple's disease (intestinal lipodystrophy): Intestinal disease caused by bacterial infection (malabsorption due to intestinal lymph flow blockage), which may also present as a systemic disease. Diagnosis made by biopsy from small intestine (PAS-positive macrophages). Eye involvement usually as part of cerebral involvement: recurrent iridocyclitis, rarely retinitis or vasculitis, occasionally also eye muscle paralysis as well as scleritis and episcleritis.

Williams (-Beuren) syndrome: Congenital cardiac defect, usually supravalvar aortic stenosis. Characteristic 'elfin' facies (small face with broad mouth), abnormal dentition, delayed mental development. Frequently strabismus, heavy upper lids, white radial streaks in the iris. Usually occurs spontaneously, but in some cases inherited as autosomal dominant with variable expression.

Wilms' tumor (nephroblastoma): Embryonic renal tumor, usually occurring by 4th year. Combination with aniridia or iris hypoplasia. WAGR syndrome.

Wilson's disease: AR-inherited disorder of copper metabolism with copper deposits. Abnormal hepatic, psychiatric, extrapyramidal and cerebellar functions. Sometimes yellow-brown Kayser-Fleischer corneal rings (copper deposition in the posterior Descemet's membrane in 90% of cases) or greenish 'sunflower' cataract. Rarely, abnormal eye movements and retinal changes.

Wolf's syndrome (partial monosomy 4p): Cardinal symptoms: antimongoloid position of lid axis, iris coloboma, broad nasal root, cleft lip and palate. Results from partial deletion of the short arm of chromosome 4.

X-chromosomal congenital retinoschisis: Central (macular) retinoschisis is characteristic. Decreased visual acuity of different degrees, usually since birth and without progression. Hyperopia is common. Half the cases have peripheral retinoschisis (usually temporal downward). Often the central retinoschisis can no longer be detected after the age of 35; instead, the number of pigment clumps in the retina is increased.

Zellweger's syndrome (cerebrohepatorenal syndrome): Abnormal peroxysomal function resulting from point mutation. AR. Multiple malformations, mental retardation with epileptic seizures, severe hypotonia of skeletal muscles and markedly abnormal liver functions. Death in infancy. Eye involvement: nystagmus, corneal clouding, cataract, anomalies of retinal vessels and of the pigment epithelium, disc defects, iridocorneal adhesions and congenital glaucoma.

INDEX